RA Rheumatoid Arthritis

Managing Rheumatoid Arthritis.

How to effectively cope with rheumatoid arthritis: pain relief, treatment, diet and remedies.

by

Robert Rymore

Table of Contents

3

Chapter 1: Introduction

Arthritis in general and Rheumatoid Arthritis (RA) in particular have stopped making headlines in the newspapers or medical journals for almost two decades now. This doesn't mean that the disease has stopped confronting people or there is somewhat less number of people being affected from it. The truth is people have accepted it as a harsh reality of life and now they are trying to deal with it. This book is aimed for people who want to make necessary adjustments in their life that can enable them to live a full life despite having RA. This book highlights the crucial connections that can lead to a normal life for anyone suffering from RA and emphasizes that this public health issue needs to be treated aggressively.

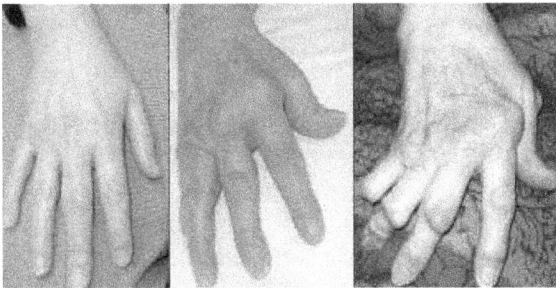

Epidemiology is the cornerstone of research in quantitative analysis of any particular disease. It examines the balance of probabilities, relates statistical data and explains the effectiveness of research methodologies. In doing these, it becomes an important tool for addressing public health issues. Many scholars have tried to define this important branch of medical science but none succeeded like John Murray Last, an emeritus professor at the University of Ottawa. He explains epidemiology as, "the study of the distribution and determinants of health-related states or events in specified populations, and the application of this study to the control of health problems". A mere glimpse on the definition tells that epidemiology of a disease can play a vital role in improving our understanding of the disease, which in turn, can better equip us to deal with it.

Scientific methods aimed at evaluating the distribution of diseases in specific human populations go a long way in improving our understanding of these diseases. When applied to chronic non-communicable diseases like RA, it can help us to make key decisions in treatment and management of RA. Now that we understand the epidemiology it is time to look at some epidemiological data related to RA. In a study published in Arthritis Rheum (2010 June) it was estimated that 1.5 million adults had rheumatoid arthritis in 2007. According to Journal of Rheumatology (2004) from 1979-1998, the annual number of arthritis and other rheumatic conditions (AORC) deaths rose from 5,537 to 9,367. RA accounts for 22% of deaths caused by AORC. While the figure of 1.5 million in 2010 is considerably less than the 1991 estimate of 2.1 million, still RA is a major health issue both on economic and physiologic fronts. At the same time, this reduction of 0.6 million suggest that better treatment options have improved the management of this disease considerably and better treatment options may further reduce its impact on our health.

Depending upon different factors, RA can manifest itself in three different pathways.

-1: Monocyclic RA. This type of episode lasts for only 3-5 years there is no subsequent recurrences. This is usually achieved through a timely diagnosis and or an aggressive treatment.

-2: Ploycyclic RA. This type involves frequent episodes of varying intensity, sometimes moderate while at other times it may be severe.

-3: Progressive RA. This is the worst type as RA continues to deteriorate and the pain threshold increases with time.

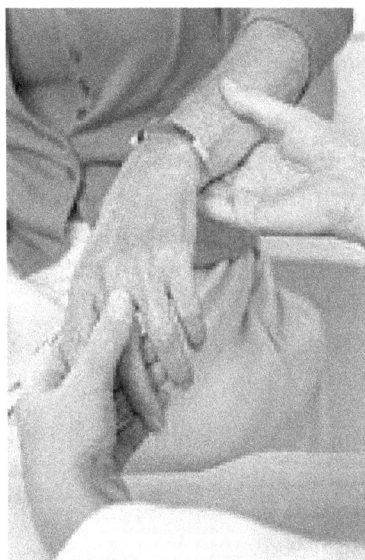

Studies suggest that 75% people diagnosed with RA are likely to experience a remission within 5 years of the diagnosis. This remission may be permanent or a recurrence may follow it. Women are more than twice as likely to suffer from RA as men. The prevalence studies showed that 9.8 out of 1000 women suffer from RA, while figure for men is only 4.1 out of 1000. The lifetime risk is 4% for women and 3% for men, further proving a female dominance in prevalence.

RA has a huge financial impact on individuals and health systems. The total costs associated with RA are almost twice the costs of osteoarthritis. This shows that RA has a more severe financial impact than osteoarthritis. Although the latest cost studies are not available for RA, but those performed in 1990's found the annual medical costs to be approximately 5673$ and indirect non-medical expenditures to be approximately 2785$. Now if we analyze these figures in the context of current economic situation and the inflation US markets have experienced in the last two decades, the cost figures will be staggering, to say the least. Rochester Epidemiology Project, a prevalence study, found that people with RA were approximately six times more likely than people without arthritis to incur medical charges, independent of RA. Another study places the lifetime (25 years after diagnosis) costs of RA at a staggering 122,000 US $.

National Institute of Arthritis & Musculoskeletal & Skin Diseases states that RA patients are 40% more likely to report poor general health as compared to people without arthritis. This poor health status is a direct result of functional loses RA patients suffer in majority of domains like work, recreational activities and social relations. Despite a relatively low prevalence, the functional disabilities are high enough to place RA as the 19th most common cause of years lost to disability.

This book will closely examine the impact of RA on the life of patients and suggest meaningful pragmatic approaches to tackle different problems they face. Emphasis will be on different treatment options available to treat it aggressively. A conscious approach has been adopted throughout the book to help readers differentiate among some very similar conditions such as systemic lupus erythematosus, psoriatic arthritis, and gout. To facilitate this simple differential diagnosis charts and images are frequently used. Technical guidelines provided by the American College of Rheumatology in THE 2010 ACR-EULAR Classification criteria for RA are explained in simple terms for non-medical audience. We hope that this book will provide the ultimate guidance a RA patient so desperately needs. Evidence based discussions will help you make necessary decisions for controlling symptom severity and achieve remission. It will also help you in identifying individual positive and negative key determinants of RA to improve your quality of life.

A) What are Auto-Immune diseases?

Autoimmune diseases are a group of nearly 100 diseases that are caused by an attack of body's own immune system on different organs, tissues and cells. Fortunately, most of the diseases in this group are rare. Unfortunately, as a group they are significant enough to disturb the lives of 14.7 to 23.5million people in the USA – up to 8% of the population. More disturbing is the fact that their prevalence is on the rise. According to the Autoimmune Diseases Coordinating Committee (ADCC) of the U.S. National Institutes of Health, most of these diseases have no absolute cures, so major efforts in research should be focused on improving the quality of life of the patients by reducing the impact of autoimmune diseases.

A better understanding of the fundamental biologic principles underlying disease onset and progression is key to finding best solutions for the patients suffering from autoimmune diseases like Rheumatoid Arthritis. Both general public and medical professionals need to be better educated about these diseases. This will check the rising prevalence. The importance of better professional education is further magnified when we consider the diverse clinical manifestations involved in autoimmune diseases. Additionally, autoimmune diseases share many features, both at their onset and during follow-up, with a number of other diseases. All these factors make it more difficult and challenging for physicians to tackle it effectively.

At the same time, despite the diverse nature of clinical manifestations of autoimmune diseases, they share a number of underlying mechanisms with other diseases. Therefore, they may respond to the conventional treatments for those diseases. In the Sixth International Congress of Autoimmunity held in Porto, Portugal, on September 2008 emphasis was drawn on the accurate diagnosis of the autoimmune diseases for successful management.

Autoimmune diseases are divided in two subgroups:

-A. Systemic Autoimmune Diseases

-B. Organ Specific Autoimmune Diseases

As we focus on Rheumatoid Arthritis which is a systemic autoimmune disease, we will describe a few organ specific autoimmune diseases in the following paragraphs briefly.

-1. Hashimoto Thyroiditis: It is one of the most frequent autoimmune diseases specific to thyroid gland. It is characterized by lymphocytic infiltration of the gland resulting in either loss of function or hyperthyroidism.

-2. Atrophic Thyroiditis: Also specific to thyroid gland, this autoimmune disorder is characterized by antibodies targeting the gland. Other physiological markers include functional hypothyroidism and absence of goiter.

-3. Sub-Acute Thyroiditis: More commonly referred to as giant cell thyroiditis or pseudogranulomatous thyroiditis, it is characterized by severe pain in the gland which may be due to association of a variety of viral infections. These infections don't have any direct role in the pathogenesis (The origin and development of a disease or the mechanism whereby something causes a disease) of Sub-Acute Thyroiditis.

-4. Graves' disease: Another thyroid specific autoimmune disease associated with the production of specific antibodies that produce toxic effect on the gland.

-5. Postpartum Thyroiditis: The hormonal changes in women after delivery are supposed to be responsible for this autoimmune disease. These women do have normal thyroid functions prior to the conception.

-6. Autoimmune Diabetes Mellitus: It is a cellular autoimmune disorder targeting the pancreatic cells that produce insulin. In this disorder beta cells (insulin producers) of pancreas are targeted by the immune system.

-7. Autoimmune Adrenalitis: Also known as Autoimmune Addison's Disease, Autoimmune adrenalitis was considered a rare disease in the 70's but since then its prevalence has increased threefold. Major clinical manifestations include adrenal failure and loss of enzymes.

-8. Autoimmune Hypophysitis: An immune-mediated inflammation of the pituitary gland, this autoimmune disease damages the gland tissue and if untreated my lead to pituitary dysfunction.

-9. Autoimmune Parathyroid Disease: the mechanism of the disease is not completely understood and it is supposed to be cell mediated response to parathyroid antigens.

-10. Autoimmune Polyendocrine Syndromes: A group of diseases involving multiple gland failures in the endocrine system involving organ specific antibodies.

-11. Endometriosis: 10-47% women undergoing infertility surgery are likely to develop this autoimmune disorder. Pain and infertility represent the major clinical problems of women with endometriosis.

-12. Autoimmune Ovarian Failure: It is associated with autoimmune pathologies like the one in Addison's disease. The immune system attack may be global or specific to ovarian antibodies.

-13. Autoimmune Orchitis: The mechanism of disease in autoimmune orchitis is unknown and probably involves the access of the immune system to the testis due to inflammation, infection, or trauma in response to antigens or microorganisms. Approximately 10% infertile men are affected by this disease.

-14. Other Common Organ Specific Autoimmune Disorders:

-a: Autoimmune Hepatitis

-b: Primary Biliary Cirrhosis

-c: Primary Sclerosing Cholangitis

-d: Autoimmune Pancreatitis

-e: Autoimmune Gastritis

-f: Ulcerative Colitis

-g: Inflammatory Bowel Disease

-h: Celiac Disease

-i: Pemphigus and Bullous Pemphigoid

-j: Vitiligo

-k: Autoimmune Dilated Cardiomyopathy

-l: Rheumatic Fever

-m: Idiopathic Interstitial Pneumonias

-n: Pulmonary Arterial Hypertension

-o: Multiple Sclerosis

-p: Paraneoplastic Neurological Syndromes

-q: Neuromylelitis Optica (Devic Syndrome)

-r: Autoimmune Epilepsy

B) Defining rheumatoid arthritis

Arthritis is a Greek word derived from two words. "Arthron" means joints and Latin"-itis" means inflammation. Actually the word is used to explain a variety of different joint disorders.

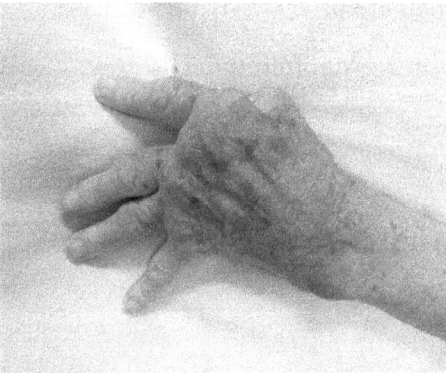

Arthritis has many different types with different routes of inflammation causing damage to joints. Some types are not caused by inflammation at all. Rheumatoid arthritis (RA) is a type of inflammatory arthritis. It is defined as:

"It is characterized by chronic pain and joint destruction, premature mortality and an elevated risk of disability, with high

costs for those suffering from this disease and for society. If this condition is not treated, joint destruction from bone erosion can be expected, as well as progressive inabilities, leading eventually to disability, after a time period that can vary from only a few months to many years, depending on prognostic factors."

RA usually affects the small joints of the hands and the feet, and typically both sides equally, although any synovial joint can be affected. As it is a systemic disease, it can affect the whole body, including the heart, lungs and eyes.

Awareness is one thing which is sorely missed among RA patients. They need to be better equipped with latest information about the disease. As the last two decades saw a decrease in overall prevalence through better management and treatment options available to the RA patients. This trend suggests that better awareness campaigns can further reduce the RA prevalence and impact. Patients must have understanding of what actually rheumatoid arthritis is, how it affects, and what to do for management and cure of the disease. If family members and care givers know better about this disease, its potential complications and treatment available to them, only then they can better provide support to patients. Moreover, patients will be able to communicate better with health care professionals resulting in improved

The name is historically based on "rheumatic fever", sickness which consists of joint pain and is derived from the Greek word εὐμα-rheuma (nom.), εὐματος-rheumatos (gen.) ("flow, current"). The -oid ("resembling") gives the meaning as joint inflammation that look like rheumatic fever.

One school of notion is that RA is a disease of the recent age and its pathogenesis is an outcome of an environmental or genetic stimulus that was not in ancient times. According to second theory RA existed in ancient people but had never been well characterized.

By going through studies and research conducted in different eras, it is concluded that

- RA is not a disease of modern origin, and was both present perhaps thousands of years ago.

- RA occurs as a response to an environmental stimulus or stimuli experienced by genetically vulnerable individuals.

- The uniqueness and origins of these stimuli or provocative events are still not known completely although tempting signs have appeared.

- Distinct environmental activators may be important in detachment of patients with RA. For example, smoking may be a major risk factor in RA patients who carry an MHC allele that encodes the common epitope and that has auto antibodies to proteins containing citrulline. Therefore the historical investigation of RA we now define as RA is more than one disease.

Chapter 2: **Joints in Rheumatoid Arthritis**

The human skeleton consist of more than one hundred joints. Many of these joints move very slightly or not at all, and we are mostly not aware of them. Different types of joints work in diverse ways to attain different functions.

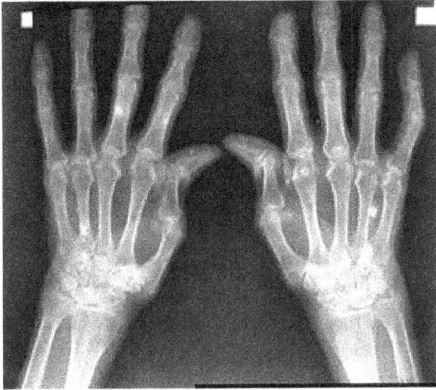

The joints can be divided into three basic types depending on amount of motion each allows. These are:

- Rigid (Skull and pelvis>> not affected in RA).

- Slightly mobile (vertebrae in the spine joints >>not affected in RA).

- Freely movable (shoulders, elbows, wrists, finger and toe joints, hips, knees, and ankles >>affected by RA).

Inflammation of the joints and tissue around joints are characteristic features of rheumatoid arthritis. When taking into account how RA affects the joints and why it creates some of the symptoms, it is significant to know that no two people with RA are just alike. The severity of RA differs from one individual to other and joint to joint. Because of these differences it is often difficult to judge exactly how much joint damage the disease has caused.

15

A) Inflammation

Our body has a natural defense mechanism to fight against infection, illness and disease. Inflammation occurs when our bodies experience any damage as a response to injury or infection. Inflammation is part of the body's immune system response to the injury or infection. The signs and symptoms of inflammation are warmth, pain, redness, and swelling. Inflammation is self-limiting and the amount of inflammation involved usually depends on the severity of the injury or infection. Under normal conditions, cells of immune system like unique white blood cells called lymphocytes, neutrophils and macrophages tactically interact with one another to achieve controlled inflammation.

B) Difference between Inflammation of RA and Normal Inflammation

The inflammation in RA involves the white cells described above, but the initiating event or the cause of this inflammation is unknown. This trigger or activator could be a virus or another foreign substance or antigen (anything that is foreign to body). In general, antigens are removed and smashed by the body's immune system. Some theories suggest that it is this process that goes wrong in RA. When a defensive cell called the macrophage catches up to the antigen it stimulates an increase in the number of two types of lymphocytes that is T and B cells. Normally they have an integral but self-limiting role in fighting infections. In RA these cells become chronically "agitated," and this agitation works to maintain inflammation in the joints. Continued inflammation produces the heat, swelling, and pain due to excessive blood accumulation at the site of inflammation.

When no known antigen is present, the body appears to fight against itself. Therefore, RA is often called an autoimmune disease in which Immune cells mistakenly react against the body's own healthy cells, causing inflammation. Patients suffering from autoimmune diseases have antibodies in their blood that attack their own body tissues, which can lead to inflammation.

C) Causes

The cause of rheumatoid arthritis is unknown. But some factors may be considered as causative:

Infectious agents

Although infectious agents such as viruses, bacteria and fungi have long been suspected, but not a single one has proven as a definitive cause yet.

Genetic factors

This possible cause of rheumatoid arthritis is a very active research area worldwide. It is believed that the affinity to develop rheumatoid arthritis may be genetically inherited (hereditary). Certain genes have been identified that increase the risk for rheumatoid arthritis.

Environmental factors

Environmental factors also sometime seem to play a role in causing rheumatoid arthritis. For example, scientists have reported that smoking tobacco, exposure to some minerals of silica, and chronic periodontal disease, enhance the risk of developing rheumatoid arthritis.

Certain infections or factors in the environment might trigger the activation of the immune system in susceptible individuals. This abnormal immune system then attacks the body's own tissues which lead to inflammation in the joints and sometimes in different organs of the body, such as the lungs or eyes etc.

In spite of all this information the exact trigger is still unknown. Currently the only confirmed cause of RA is the self-attacking immune system that is activated to produce inflammation in the joints and infrequently other tissues of the body. Immune cells, called lymphocytes, are activated and chemical messengers (cytokines, like tumor necrosis factor/TNF, interleukin-1/IL-1, and interleukin-6/IL-6) are appeared in the inflamed areas.

D) PATHOGENESIS (the origination and development of a disease)

Rheumatoid arthritis is an autoimmune disease that is linked with progressive disability, systemic problems, and an early death. Although the origination part of rheumatoid arthritis is unknown, however, progress in understanding the development of the disease has created severalnew therapeutic pathways for successful treatment.

E) The Stages of RA or Disease progression

RA can be divided into five stages. Each stage is characterized by the category of the uncontrolled inflammation in the joints.

Stage 1

In first stage, person with RA has no symptoms of arthritis, and their joints appear normal. Some of these people may be genetically susceptible to arthritis. Presence of RA gene marker alone is not enough to cause someone to develop RA, however. It is supposed that some unknown trigger actually begins the progression of arthritis in the genetically susceptible person; i.e., exogenous factor, likely an infectious organism, targets the synovia and elicits a chronic immune response and other unknown factors maintain it by blocking normal declaration of the inflammation. According to one theory in RA, the communication between cells is disturbed by some way, permitting inflammation to persist for long periods of time.

Stage 2

This is the stage during which first symptoms of RA appear. Early in the path of arthritis, small lymphocytes move into the synovial membranes, resulting in condition called as synovitis, or inflammation of the synovium .The macrophages and lymphocytes keep on promoting inflammation by producing cytokines, "chemical messengers" which are responsible for carrying messages from one part of the body toanother.

Two particular cytokines, tumor necrosis factor (TNF) and interleukin-1 (IL-1) have been recognized as inflammation accelerators. People with RA have large amount of TNF and IL-1 in their joints. Cytokines can provoke an increase in the number of blood vessels going to the synovium, and with amplified blood flow, the joints become warm. The seepage of cytokines into the blood stream may also cause feeling of fatigue that is so common in RA. Other cytokines are, to some extent, responsible for stimulating cells to produce prostaglandins and leukotrienes, both of which are effective producers of inflammation. Sustained production of cytokines, prostaglandins, leukotrienes, and other substances directly contribute to swelling, heat, and pain in the joints.

Another important event in the development of RA is the transformation of B lymphocytes into another type of white blood cells, the plasma cells, which produce antibodies. Antibodies, also called as immune-globulins, are unique proteins that the body normally manufactures to fight against viruses and foreign bacteria, and are not normally present in the body. In RA, for reasons that are indistinct, the bodies appear to produce an extreme amount of antibodies. One particular antibody often found in the blood of people with RA is called the "rheumatoid factor". The production of rheumatoid factor worsens the inflammatory process.

Stage 3

In this stage there is a noticeable rise in the number of cells in the synovium, possibly provoked by the presence of various cytokines. The synovium becomes greatly thicker, or hypertrophied, and this makes the joint feel soft or spongy. An increase in the amount of synovial fluid in the joint causes stiffness and restriction of motion of the joints. (Gathering of joint fluid is known as joint effusion). There is also an increase in hyaluronic acid, the lubricating material in the synovial joint fluid. Many people consider that large amount of hyaluronic acid is responsible for morning rigidity or stiffness and the rigidity experienced after sitting for a prolonged period of time without moving is gelling phenomenon).

Normally Joint fluid has inflammatory white blood cells called neutrophils or polymorpho-nuclear leukocytes. In the joint affected by RA, neutrophils unite lymphocytes in enabling the inflammatory process. In testing for RA, the physician may remove a sample of fluid from the joints to resolve the relative proportions of these cells present. This helps the physician to differentiate RA from other types of arthritis.

A person may experience major joint symptoms including pain, heat, swelling, stiffness, and limited motion in either second or third stage of RA. All of these inflammatory changes are potentially reversible with appropriate medical therapy.

Stage 4

At this stage, swollen synovium can mature or proliferate, scattering on the top of joint cartilage. When synovium grows up as such, it is called "pannus".

The pannus secretes enzymes called collagenases, which can destroy collagen (cartilage proteins). Joint fluid has Neutrophils that can also discharge harmful enzymes. There are many other useful enzymes in the body, these specific enzymes can degrade the cartilage that guards the bones and joints.

Collagenases can also cause the bone to break down in the area in which the synovia joins together with bone. Outcome of this is the formation of small openings or erosions in the bone and cartilage. Erosions commonly occur first at the point where protecting cartilage ends at the boundaries of joints.

Stage 5

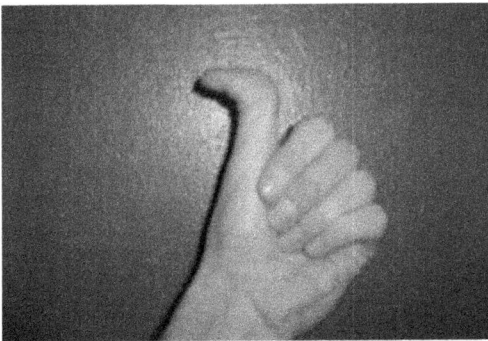

The pannus can further attack and corrode through cartilage and bone by producing more enzymes if the arthritis is left untreated. Any malfunctioning of cartilage decreases the amount of support between the bones of the joint. When cartilage is scraped by this erosion, the capacity to have smooth joint movement or activity is lost. People with RA can feel a rasping feeling in the joint during movement, and physicians can also feel the grating of the joint during physical assessment. This rasping is called "crepitus".

Continuous breakdown of cartilage leads tototally gnarled cartilage by pannus. So in stage 5 of RA, abandoned swelling can cause ligaments and tendons to widen, causing the shakiness of the joint. Muscles become smaller and weaker due to damage (atrophy) because of neglect. Stretched ligaments and tendons and atrophied muscles obstruct with the joint's ability to function appropriately, often causing joint to not move as it was intended to.

21

Inflammation and pannus can extend along the tendons in tenosynovitis, making the tendons feeble and thus causing greater risk for rupture. When the cartilage become craggy and the supporting structures are disrupted, other alterations sometime occur which change the former shape and function of the joint. These mechanical changes occur as a result of more abnormal forces produced by erosions and changes in shape of cartilage. They also prolong and deteriorate the inflammation in joints.

Later in this stage, after the complete erosion of cartilage, the amount of inflammation and swelling frequently decreases, producing conditions which are sometimes called as burnt out joints. At this stage the lengthened ligaments and tendons can in fact become even weaker, as the swelling approaching against them is reducing. The slackness of these sustaining structures can critically affect the constancy of the joint.

Chapter 3: Symptoms & Diagnosis

Initially patient may observe discomfort in some joints like fingers, knuckles, wrists and or the balls of feet. Usually, RA is a 'symmetrical' arthritis which means it influences both wrists and both hands in the same way. Symptoms of disease vary from person to person. For some, RA develops somewhat slowly at first. Other people discover the state comes on rapidly and painfully, making it hard to carry out every day activities.

Symptoms include:

- Stiffness in the morning, or if patient doesn't change posture for a long time

- Pain and swelling surrounding the joints, making them red and warm,

- Reduced hold potency,

- Weariness, that can lead to feelings of irritability and despair.

Symptoms outside the joints include:

- Flu like symptoms such as fever,

- Weight loss,

- Inflammation in the eyes,

- Rheumatoid nodules,

- Inflammation of other body parts like lungs, blood, blood vessels andthe membrane surrounding heart (rarely)

A) Stiffness

Joint stiffness can affect any joint, but most commonly affected joints are of hands, feet, hips, knees, and spine. The joint is difficult to use and might have a restricted sort of motion.

Morning stiffness is one of the characteristic symptoms of rheumatoid arthritis. While many people with suffering from other forms of arthritis have stiff joints in the morning, it takes people with rheumatoid arthritis from an hour to several hours sometimes to get rid of the morning fitness.

The cause of morning stiffness from RA is not completely clear, but there is a series of reaction that goes something like as:

Joint inflammation first cause swelling in the joint, which later increases,once the joint becomes motionless. This swelling can cause contraction of muscles around the joints. It is a common sense that the stiffness is often poorer when the joint has been at rest for long time like while sleeping or sitting for a long time. This stiffness gets better with activity.

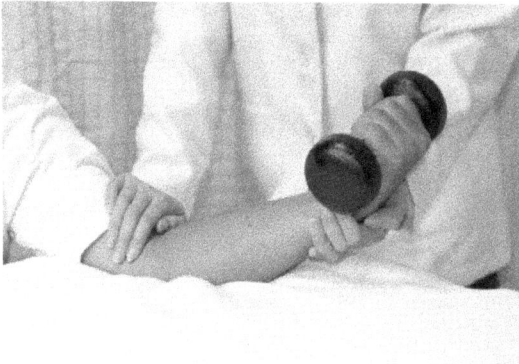

Reducing RA Stiffness

One should follow following strategies to get relief from stiffness:

- Begin with mild movements,
- Keep yourself warm,
- Take few minutes of exercise,
- Applying joint cream,
- Take adequate vitamin D and calcium,
- Confer with therapist.

B) Pain and Swelling

Inflammation in a joint makes it sensitive and weak. Lengthened inflammation causes deteriorationandaggravate pain. Rheumatoid arthritis (RA) is a disease that damages the lining and cartilage of the joints. This results in painful swelling. It can cause eternal damage, so appropriate and early treatment is essential.

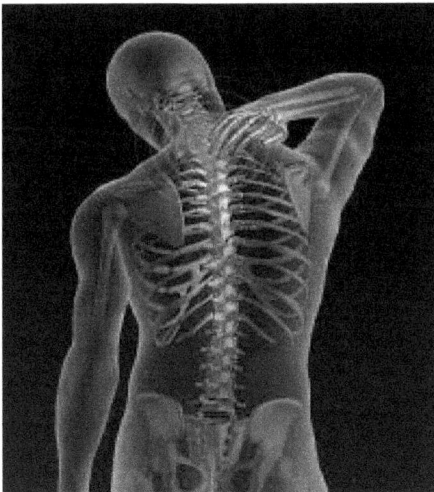

Pain and swelling is multifaceted and the causes of pain in RA may be due to inflammation and/or associated mechanical factors so combination of treatment is required.

Following strategies can be applied to get relief from pain:

- Resting inflamed joints
- Use of splints in site.

- Applying heat or cold to painful joints
- Hot baths or showers can ease stiff joints
- Exercise
- Drug therapy.
- Joint replacement therapy in case of severe damage to joints.

C) Symptoms related to other parts

Blood and blood vessels - - Blood

RA affects the blood in such a way that the number of red blood cells decreases remarkably. Anemia may develop as one of the consequences of continued inflammation, and its harshness often reflects the severity of the arthritis. It is called the "anemia of chronic disease".This type of anemia usually gets better when the arthritis is properly controlled.

In some conditions, the drug erythropoietin is administered intravenously to augment red blood cell production for the time being. This medication can be used in a pre-surgical condition.

Another type of anemia, known as "iron deficiency anemia", may also develop as a side effect of taking non-steroidal anti-inflammatory drugs, which can infuriate the stomach lining and cause minor and sometime major loss of blood via ulceration. So in this situation it may be essential to stop non-steroidal anti-inflammatory drug (NSAID) therapy and to start a course of stomach healing medicines.

Blood vessels

Inflammation of blood vessels, known as vasculitis, is a rare complication of RA that usually affects individuals who have high level of rheumatoid factor in their blood.

Blood vessels may develop inflammation when antibody production by plasma cells increases in blood. The antibodies stick to each other and form complexes,these floating immune complexes occasionally deposit themselves on the blood vessel wall, resulting in limiting the flow of blood and causing inflammation within the blood vessels.

Depending on the size and location of the affected blood vessels, vasculitis can be a comparatively minor problem or a more significant one.

- Skin ulcers may develop when small blood vessels going to the skin are involved. Crack like lesions around and beneath the finger nails can occur. These ulcers and lesions usually require only scrupulous skin care to stop a possible infection of the skin. By using mild antiseptic soap, carefully washing/drying the skin and then using sterile bandage over it can beenough for prevention.

- Affected blood vessels leading to the nerves make them weak as well. This may lead to neuropathy.

- More often vasculitis may involve the larger blood vessels that project to internal organs. When nerves or internal organs are affected by vasculitis, very burly medications, including corticosteroidsand cyclophosphamide, are used to treat the state and stop further damage to nerves and organs.

Eyes and Mouth

About 15 % of people with RA build up sicca syndrome. That involves dry mouth, dry eyes, or both. Occasionally the eyelids turn red and irritated.A dry, windy atmosphere or exposure to air conditioning can make the symptoms worse.

Eyes

Certain kinds of cold medications like sleep inducing medications, tranquilizers, and muscle relaxants can all increase eye dryness in RA. It can be prevented by use of eye lubricants and immediately going to physicians

An ophthalmologistcan examine a person to find the presence of either of the two other conditions in RA. These are "scleritis" and "episcleritis", they must be treated.

Mouth

Dryness of mouth may also occur in RA by inflammation of the salivary glands. Side effects of many medications can worsen the problem of dry mouth.

Excellent oral hygiene is vital, because a decrease in saliva can prompt tooth decay. Use of antiseptic mouthwash, brushing with tartar control toothpaste numerous times a day will provide protection against decay. It is also important to avoid candies. New treatments are presented that cause the salivary glands to secrete saliva. These are pilocarpine (Salagen) and cevimeline (Evoxac). Consult doctor in case of severe problem.

Skin

- Patients, in general, first observe skin nodules often close to joints in areas like tendons or in bony positions such as elbows, knuckles or Achilles. That appear under the skin as small loops called rheumatoid nodules, and they occur in about one fourth of people with developed RA mostly in those having rheumatoid factor.

- The nodules are troublesome only when they press against inner body structures. .Rheumatoid nodules are not painful unless they are positioned in an area that is frequently traumatized, such as the heel tendon, which is rubbed by the back of the shoe.

- Rheumatoid nodules infrequently appear in places other than the skin. Such as in the lungs, heart, eyes, and vocal cord. Sometimes they accompany symptoms and at other times there are no symptoms.

- Rheumatoid nodules do not require special treatment unless they cause pain, decrease function, or become infected. But presence of nodules may point to a more severe form of arthritis. Treatment with DMARDs can cause decrease of nodules and also add to some improvement. In more severe cases surgical removal is also recommended to improve the appearance.

The Heart

The heart is rarely affected in RA, and even when it does most people don't experience symptoms.

Pericarditis occur when inflammation of pericardium (membrane surrounding heart) take place. Symptoms may be similar to that of pleurisy. Pericardial effusion occurs also when considerable amount of fluid accumulates in and surrounding the heart.

Treatment involves the use of corticosteroids and only infrequently requires drainage of the fluid.

Chest and Lungs

- RA can create breathing distress in 2 ways.

1) The first when the joints between the collar bones (clavicles) and chest bone (sternum) build up arthritis. About 30 percent of people with RA develop this situation, this also cause pain when deep breaths are taken or with the movement of shoulders. The situation gets better with treatment of the arthritis.

2) Secondly when inflammation in pleura (the lining around the lungs) occurs. This fluid around the lungs generally produces few symptoms, and its presence is identified only by x-ray.

- Temporary treatment is with oral corticosteroids.

- Rheumatoid nodules may develop in the lungs which are similar to those in skin. They generally cause no symptoms and are diagnosed only by x-ray.

- A biopsy of the nodule may be required to decide its cause.

- Cough and shortness of breath are signs that pneumonitismay exist because of inflammation of lung tissue. In this case anti-inflammatory medications are directed to decrease inflammation and stop scaring.

The Bones

Osteoporosis is major condition that people with RA develop. Osteoporosis is thinning of the bones in which bone mass gradually decreasesrendering patient more susceptible to fractures. According to researchers inflammation plays a chief role in the development of osteoporosis even in early stages of RA.

How RA leads to osteoporosis is not very difficult to understand .Pro-inflammatory cytokines activate a protein called osteoprotegerin. This protein stimulates the action of a group of cells called osteoclasts that are well known for their capacity to break down bone. Some bone loss by osteoclast is normal on a daily basis in everyone but increased loss can cause permanent damage and eventually lead to osteoporosis.

Women are at elevated risk of osteoporosis than men, because they start with less initial bone mass because of menopause in which bone loss speeds up significantly. Men with RA are not safe completely from this condition, however. In addition to the direct effects of RA on bone, other changes may occur. Men with RA can have decreased levels of testosterone, which can cause extra bone loss and osteoporosis.

Other reason are:

- Arthritis medications may also increase the chance for osteoporosis such as corticosteroids are the most common cause of drug induced bone loss.

- Life style such as smoking and use of heavy alcohol is toxic to bone.

- Avoiding weight bearing exercises increase a person's risk of developing osteoporosis.

- Clacium low diet and low vitamin D in diet.

D) Diagnosis

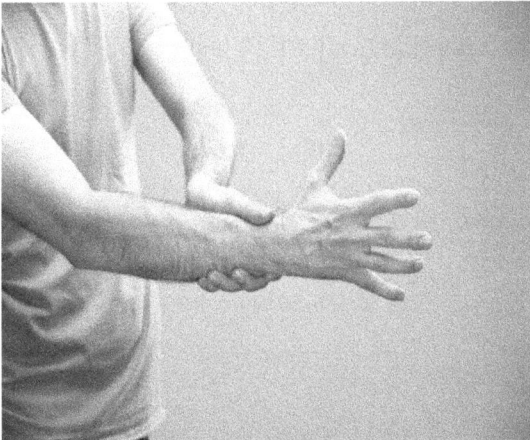

The pain of RA startssomewhat differently for every patient.There are no specific symptoms by which the doctor can confirm RA instantly.

In diagnosis following steps are involved:

-   The clinical history,
-   The physical examination,

- Differential diagnosis (involve diagnostic tests).
- Although, there are three steps involved, still it is very hard to diagnose a patient for rheumatoid arthritis straight away. Diagnostic examinations include both physical situation and medical tests. A comprehensive diagnosis comprise of following steps:
- Physical Examination (warmth, redness and swelling are observed),
- X-rays (to estimatate the progression of RA over a specific time),
- ESR Observation (Increased ESR rate calculates inflammatory process),

- Two Different Blood Tests:

(a) Rheumatoid factor (RF) diagnostic test

(b) Anti-cyclic citrullinated peptide (anti-CCP) test.

Chapter 4: Surgical treatments

Like all other medical complications, rheumatoid arthritis can cause serious pain and can create circumstances demanding radical measures. Patients have to opt for surgical treatment to restore normal health conditions. A point can be reached in illness where medication can no longer work enough and the patient is left with the only option of surgery. Good things can be said for several modern surgical treatments that work well in favor of the patients. Surgeons are putting in lot of efforts to provide improved recoveries and rehabilitation. They are doing so with the help of latest technology based surgeries that offer long lasting solutions for rheumatoid arthritis patients. However, there are many rumors and negative aspects relating to surgical treatments. We don't assume whether surgical treatments are beneficial or not. Rather, we should have a brief look at some popular treatment options to establish a better understanding ourselves. This will enable us to decide which specific surgery can benefit rheumatoid arthritis patients more.

A) Candidates for surgery

A very common situation that requires surgical operation is when pain remains severe in joints despite having all medications and complementary therapies. Although, deciding whether to have a surgery or not can be very confusing on our own. Nevertheless, a professional doctor is the right person to diagnose you to undergo any surgical procedure.

There are surgical procedures that can be successfully operated on single or multiple joints. However, there is no particular treatment that can eliminate the disease on the whole from all joints in the entire body.

B) Surgical treatment options

Types of Surgeries & their desired purposes:

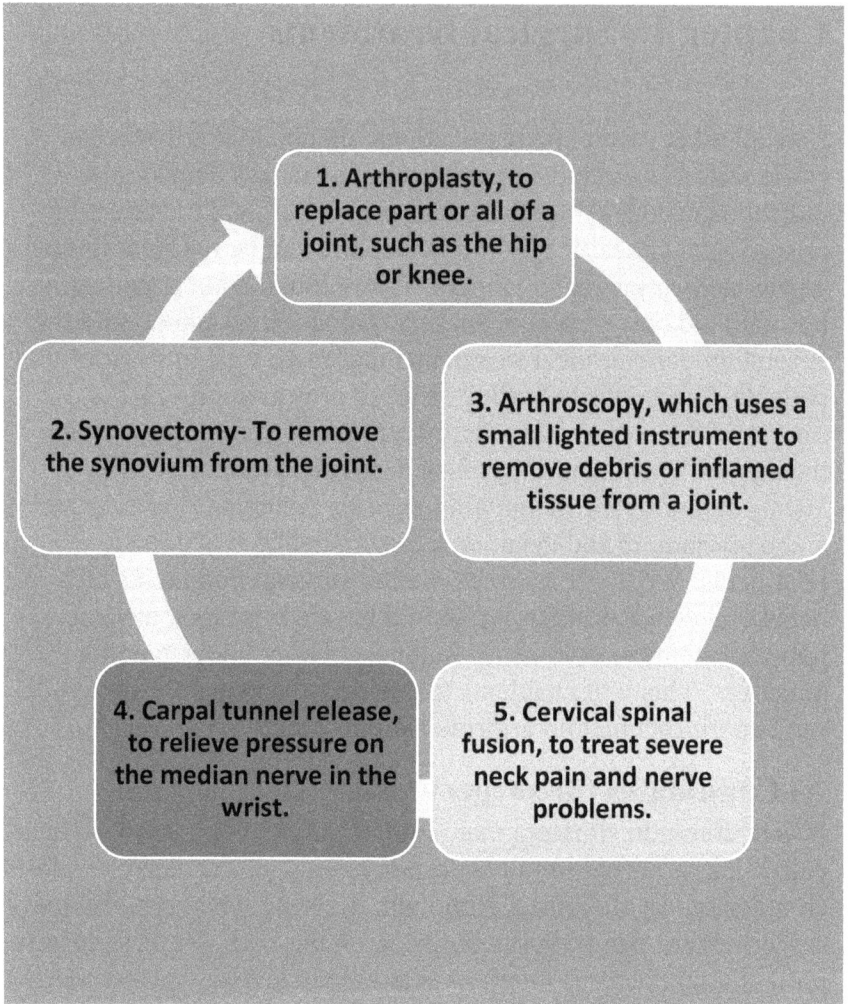

1. Arthroplasty, to replace part or all of a joint, such as the hip or knee.

2. Synovectomy- To remove the synovium from the joint.

3. Arthroscopy, which uses a small lighted instrument to remove debris or inflamed tissue from a joint.

4. Carpal tunnel release, to relieve pressure on the median nerve in the wrist.

5. Cervical spinal fusion, to treat severe neck pain and nerve problems.

Orthopedic surgeon will diagnose your situation in detail and will suggest what would be ideal for you in long term. There are different surgeries targeting specific results for rheumatoid arthritis patients. Following are some common treatments available:

1) Arthroplasty- This surgery involves joint replacement and joint restructuring in knees and hips. Deformity is responsible for severe pain and arthroplasty is a popular and effective surgery for correcting bone and joint deformations. Arthroplasty is more suitable for youngsters.

2) Arthroscopy- A particular instrument is used to remove inflamed tissues and debris from affected joints.

3) Carpal tunnel release- This surgery involves median nerve present in the wrist. The operation is carried out so that the pressure is lowered on this particular nerve to ease pain and inflammation in patients' wrist.

4) Synovectomy- It is also done to remove inflamed tissues from the joint. Synovium is removed that is responsible for excretion of chemicals that inhibits inflammation and pain in rheumatoid arthritis. There are some side-effects related to this surgery like bleeding, but it can slow down the process of disintegration of a joint significantly.

5) Finger and hand surgeries- Most of the joint problems related to hands and fingers are operated under this category.

6) Cervical spinal fusion- This surgery involves both treatment of joints and nerves causing pain in back and neck area.

7) Phalangeal head resection- Joint and nerve surgeries in the feet are termed as Phalangeal head resection. Infected joint is removed completely from the body. It is not a popular option in recent times because very few joints can be removed completely from the body.

- Handy tips for getting "Fit for Surgery"-

1. Get as much exercise as you can to improve your fitness and strengthen the muscles around your joints.

2. If you have breathing problems, such as asthma, try to make sure your chest is as good as it can be.

3. If you are overweight, try to shed some extra pounds.

4. Try to avoid infections. This includes dealing with bad or loose teeth and infected toenails.

5. If you are a woman on oral contraceptives, you may wish to stop taking them because they increase the risk of a blood clot.

Chapter 5: Natural Supplements & Home Remedies

Researchers and physicians in collaboration are exploring multiple options in conventional and natural treatments. All these efforts are aimed at helping rheumatoid arthritis patients to either get rid of all related symptoms of this specific disorder or at least minimize their pain and inflammation. Learning more about these complementary therapies and home remedies can certainly help you in living a healthier life and treat your rheumatoid arthritis more effectively. Also, do not consider these therapies as a complete recovery program rather they can only provide support towards your well-being.

A) Common dietary supplements

Historically, men and women have mostly depended upon natural ways to discover cures for various diseases and to accomplish relieve from different kinds of pain, right from the start of their existence. In the past, natural remedies and herbal medicines have always been one of the safest ways to treat *Rheumatoid arthritis* symptoms. This notion stands true in many ways even today. For thousands of years, many natural remedies have claimed to treat and sooth rheumatic pain but very few have proven their true efficacy in clinical studies against this disease. Nonetheless, omega-3 fatty acids, chondroitin and glucosamine are among few exceptions as these have truly helped in reducing rheumatoid arthritis symptoms, and alleviating pain and inflammation caused by it.

A very common problem that rheumatoid arthritis' patients have to face is that, there is a huge range of products available which might not help them in reducing their pain at all. Rather, they are more specific to other certain kinds of arthritis. So it becomes significant to make sure the effectiveness and safety of the product is proven for rheumatoid arthritis patients.

1) Glucosamine : It is a natural amino acid present in the body's cartilage. Many clinical studies have suggested that glucosamine can reduce pain and stiffness in small joints in the human body. It can be as beneficial as ibuprofen medicine. However, the positive results of the glucosamine supplements will take around two weeks to show an effect. 750 mg twice a day is recommended dose of glucosamine supplements, the supplements can be synthetic and may include shellfish extracts. Glucosamine supplements are generally more effective when taken with chondroitin. Patients that are diabetic or allergic to shellfish must take preventive measures and consult their doctor before consuming such supplements.

2) Chondroitin : It is produced in the body to increase elasticity of cartilage. Chondroitin supplements can be used to make-up for its deficiency. Chondroitin is generally made from the cow's windpipe and is also safe to try as it has no serious side-effects. 600 mg once a day is recommended dose for an ideal period of two to three months. Patients suffering from blood clotting disorder should take medical advice before taking chondroitin supplements.

3) Fish-Oils : Most of the fish oils are considered as the best source for omega-3 fatty acids. Fishes that are rich in fatty acids like DHA and EPA include halibut, mackerel, salmon, tuna and herring. Most of the nutrients in the fish oils are healthy specifically for brain improvement. Multiple trials have shown that these nutrients are also significant in controlling rheumatoid arthritis that occurs due to our own immune system malfunction. 3gm per day is recommended dose for fish-oil intake. However, 3gm of fish oil means 10-12 capsules which can be more than enough consumption for warfarin like anticoagulants. Such amount of consumption may cause minor side-effects like nose-bleeding, nausea and diarrhea.

4) Flaxseed oil: This oil contains a specific kind of omega-3 fatty acid name alpha linolenic acid (ALA).This form has the ability to be naturally converted by our body into EPA, which has proven anti-inflammatory characteristics. Flaxseed oil is not a proven food that relief's rheumatoid arthritis pain but can be used as replacement oil by those who may experience issues with fish oils. It is a natural laxative, but females with breast cancer (hormone-sensitive types) or uterine cancer should avoid it as it can interfere blood thinning.

5) Collagen:Collagen is one of those proteins that are consumed in their type II form, to relief pain from swollen joints in juvenile arthritis and rheumatoid arthritis. Type II collagen can be sourced from chicken breastbones. 60-500mcg is the recommended dose for collagen type II. Its consumption can provide soothing effect in mobility of joints.

6)Melatonin:Pineal gland in our brain is involved in the production of melatonin hormone. A hormone that is responsible for regulating our sleep patterns. Obviously, this hormone level in the blood is at maximum during the night. Although, it is not directly associated with pain relief in rheumatoid arthritis but it can ease insomnia that may occur due to pain related symptoms. Melatonin supplements are only advised when a patient is not experiencing any forms of anxiety and depression. Melatonin may cause increase of medications' effect used for the purpose of releasing anxiety or depression.

7) Gamma Linolenic Acid (GLA):As discussed previously, GLA is among those fatty acids that can help reduce pain and inflammation in joints that occur as a result of rheumatoid arthritis. Oils that are rich in GLA tends to relief morning stiffness, joint tenderness and pain in rheumatoid arthritis.1800mg is the recommended dosage of GLA supplements per day. It is better to consume primrose oil in the diet for GLA source, rather than using its supplements.

B) Herbal medicines

Herbal medicines are one of the most popular natural remedies to cure countless diseases.Clinical evidence has suggested that there are some herbs that do affect RA symptoms in a positive manner, and they do so by reducing pain and inflammation in the joints. Following are some of the more popular herbal medicines:

- *Uncariatomentosa (Cat's claw)*: Couple of studies have suggested that its bark of the root can be used as an immunity boosting remedy against inflammation. Additionally, it is also known for reducing symptoms of general arthritis and gastrointestinal disorders. Medical herbalists recommend a safe dose between 500–1,000mg (ideally in 3 doses) per day. Patients with diabetes should take precaution due to its possible interaction with hormonal and insulin drugs.

- *Cayenne (paprika)*: Cayenne, generally known as red pepper and chili pepper is a known natural remedy for several medical conditions including joint pain and stomach upsets. Our body produces endorphins that are natural pain relievers. Capsaicin present in cayenne stimulates the production of these endorphins to give soothing effect during the pain. Random placebo-controlled studies have also shown specific pain ease in rheumatoid patients.

- *Devil's claw*: It is a shrub that has claw like seedpods and its root is used in herbal medicines. Harpagosideis the active agent in this shrub and is extracted from the root.It has provenanti-inflammatory effects in trials.

- *Boswellia(Boswellia thurifera)*: An herb that produces frankincense resin, and is famous in Ayurvedic and Chinese medicine for the treatment of arthritis pain. Boswelliain combination with ashwagandha (an Indian herb) becomes more effective in reducing rheumatic pain and inflammation. 150mg is the recommended intake of boswellia extract.

- *Ginger*: Ginger is popular in South Asia for its use as traditional remedy against digestive problems as well as rheumatic pain. Ginger and garlic are mostly used as tangy spices used in cooking recipes both for taste and health purposes. Ginger also reduces inflammation in joints by minimizing leukotrienes (a chemical) production in human body that can cause swelling and pain.

C) Trace Minerals

Copper, Selenium & Magnesium : Trace minerals play a significant role in both balanced and anti-inflammatory diets. We can utilize their health benefits by consuming mineral supplements. Copper can be helpful in pain relief. Whereas, magnesium and selenium are essential in small proportions in our body as they help fight against several diseases, including heart disease, cancer and some types of arthritis also.

D) Homeopathic-Medicines

Some common homeopathic medicines that are usually prescribed in rheumatoid arthritis are:

*1) Rhustoxicodendro:*It reduces morning stiffness.

2) Apismellifica: It eases swollen and tender joints (typical in rheumatoid arthritis).

3) Causticum : A derivative of potassium compound may help people with joint patients, especially those sensitive to weather.

- Types	**Natural Supplements & Home Remedies**			
A) Common dietary supplements	1) Fish-Oils, 4) Flaxseed oil	2) Glucosamine, 5) Collagen, 7) Gamma Linolenic Acid (GLA)	3) Chondroitin, 6) Melatonin,	
B) Herbal medicines	- Uncariatomentosa (Cat's claw), - Boswellia (Boswellia thurifera)	- Cayenne (paprika), - Ginger	- Devil's claw,	
C) Trace Minerals	a) Copper	b) Selinium	c) Magnesium	
D) Homeopathic-Medicines	1) Rhustoxicodendron	2) Apismellifica	3) Causticum	

Table 1: Natural Supplements & Home Remedies chart.

Chapter 6: Bodywork/Alternative Therapies

The amazing power of human touch can ease and heal pain dramatically. Chiropractic, massage, and osteopathyhave become one of the most trusted part of healthcare.All such alternative therapies are targeted to recover musculoskeletal system, and to bring the body's equilibrium back to normal.If you want to manage your muscle stress and strain experience, then you need to take complete control of both your mind and body at the same time. Following well-known and proven practices can put you in the driving seat to drive away from any pain you may face in the life with rheumatoid arthritis.

A) Chiropractic

The functional relation of spinal cord with rest of the body is mainly focused in chiropractic therapy. A Canadian Daniel David Palmer was the founder of this therapy as a profession back in 1895. He explained that our body has its own built-in healing system to recover from all diseases. This healing is controlled and monitored by our nervous system. In-light of his beliefs, joints and spine in human body can experience sub-luxations or misalignments, resulting in potential painful complaints and disorders. This therapy can be an option for those facing severe back and joint pain.

B) Osteopathy

The main focus of the therapy is again on the spine and joints, just like chiropractic therapy. In 1874, a famous American physician Andrew Taylor was the first to introduce osteopathy message. This treatment is equally beneficial for adults and children. An osteopathic expert can use high velocity thrusts, manipulation techniques mixed with simpler and gentler strokes on soft tissues. Osteopaths are also highly qualified and well trained in their respective field to expertly attend rheumatoid arthritis patients on a right scale.

C) Exercise

Brain chemicals also known as neurotransmitters are produced in human brain as a result of exercise. These feelings of euphoria (produced in result of neurotransmitters) are helpful in coping with emotional stress. An evidence-based medical journal published in PubMed claimed that 15min exercise per day can enable a human being to live 3 years longer on average, reduce their mental stress and physical pain. Exercise can impose stamina and fitness to counter both physical strain and mental stress, both at work and at home.

D) Rolfing

Please note that it is not a treatment method suitable for managing rheumatic pain. Rolfing is not discussed here as a pain relieving technique, rather it is meant to discuss as a warning (to keep the patients with rheumatoid arthritis away). A type of massage that can ease the muscle tension to heal several disorders, recover health and reduce pain. However, there is no proven evidence of its direct effect on rheumatic pain In fact; Rolfing may lead to joint damage in patients with rheumatoid arthritis. For patients with symptoms of other types of arthritis it is certainly helpful in managing headaches, back pain and body stiffness.

E) Massage

Currently, there are over 80 different messages techniques in practice around the world. Obviously, basics are the same, to reduce pain, stress and maintain chemical balance. Such balance ensures hormonal stability to minimize stress, pain and restore natural immune system of the human body.

Swedish massage: Involves kneading (petrissage) or Rhythmic stroking (effleurage) of muscles & soft tissues; may include oils or electrical stimulation devices.

Chair massage: Manipulation in a specially designed chair that bends your body to improve the practitioner's access to your tense joints.

Massage Therapies (Soft Tissue Message):

Myofascial release:

Slow, gentle manipulation of your fascia—the thin tissues surrounding muscles—to stretch your tense tissues & relieve pain & stress.

Deep tissue massage:

Releases tension in deeper layers of Soft tissue than Swedish massage, with manipulation across the grain of your muscle; it also may break up scar tissue within the soft tissues.

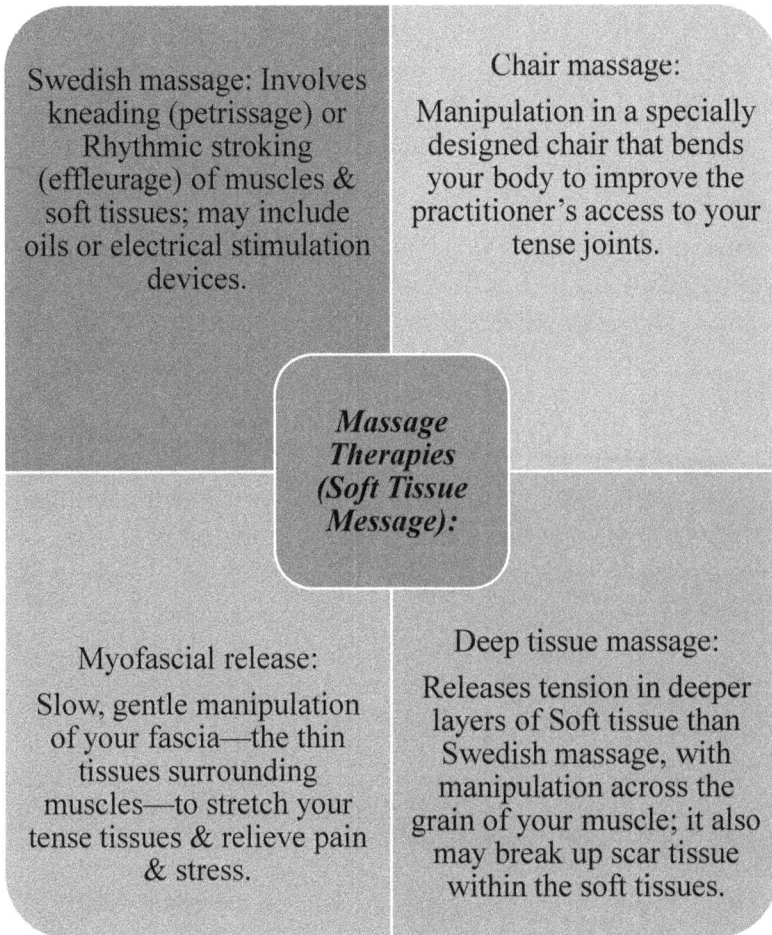

Figure 1: Soft-tissue massage-Therapies.

Massage is one the oldest and most practiced type of complementary therapy. Nevertheless, Per Henrik Ling of Sweden in nineteenth century redeveloped some of the massage techniques. That is why, it is also known as Swedish massage. Somehow, Per Henrik Ling techniques are also considered as rip-snorting (violent-using slam-bang methods). In most recent times, there are multiple soft-tissue massage techniques available that are equally helpful in pain management of rheumatoid arthritis.

F) Acupuncture

This physical therapy points to 365 crucial points in our body. It enables free flow of positive energy in our body to relax muscles and reduce physical and mental strain.

G) Yoga

Is a breathing technique with sequel movements to gain control over mind and body with relaxation point of view. Gentle movements and easy breathing postures are aimed to relief stress.

H) Reiki

There are dozens of effective spiritual-healing procedures and reiki is one of them. Its actual origin is Japan. It is similar to massage as a reiki practitioner will use a gentle touch to facilitate a flow of energy inside the body. In reiki, some practices also exclude any physical contact at all.

Chapter 7: **Inflammation in Rheumatoid Patients**

Rheumatoid arthritis is an inflammatory condition and there is direct relation between our health and food we eat or alternatively, between food and disease. Eating the right food at right time can lower the risk of many diseases that may occur as a result of inflammation. Different diet plans are for several diseases. These are based on the common concept that continuous inflammation or inflammation that is out of control in the body cause serious health problems, and that taking in food to avoid persistent inflammation encourage good health and can combat with disease.So anti inflammation diet reduces inflammation and not intended for weight loss but provide energy and sufficient vitamins, minerals,dietary fiber, essential fatty acids anddefensive phytonutrients etc. It is actually a life style that includes eating accurate, exercise, sufficient and quality sleep and stress managing.

A) Inflammation: What's the Big Deal?

There are trillion of cells present in human body. Human body will remain healthy if these cells function properly and if there will be any abnormality in these cells body fails to function properly and we will become sick.

The outer most layer of cell is cell membrane. It is most important part of the cell, made up of a lipid layer with proteins embedded in it that serve as channels for transport. Receptors are also present on cell membrane that receive signals for different molecules like amino acids, vitamins, minerals and hormones and then start a series of reactions needed by body. Import and export of information and substances must be as per requirement of the body for proper functioning.

When cells become inflamed the signal on the receptors becomes poor to the communication and further more impairment of these receptors can shut down their performance. So balance of different process across the cell become disturbed which make the cell toxic. Different organelles within the cell are infected also. For example when this problem occur with mitochondria it affects cellular energy present in the form of ATP which is necessary for cells and body to perform different function. Similarly problem in Golgi bodies can cause disturbance in secretion of some important molecules etc.

When our cells become chronically inflamed they can undergo two processes. First, they can mutate and after that can become cancerous cells. Secondly, they will die and when cells die excessively it is called aging because now the cells regulatory mechanisms are disturbed because of alterations in gene expression.

All these mentioned processes of inflammation produce symptoms, and can lead to disease progression with the passage of time, such as heart diseases, thyroid syndrome, hormonal disturbances, diabetes, autoimmune conditions and neurological problems etc.

B) Inflammation& its Types

Our body has a natural defense mechanism to fight against infections, illness and disease. Inflammation occurs when our bodies experience any damage as a response to injury or infection. Inflammation is in fact part of the body's immune system response to the injury or infection. The signs and symptoms of inflammation are warmth, pain, redness, and swelling. Inflammation is self-limiting and the amount of inflammation involved usually depends on the severity of the injury or infection. Under normal conditions, cells of immune system like unique white blood cells called lymphocytes, neutrophils and macrophages tactically interact with one another to achieve controlled inflammation.

Inflammation is sometime known as the silent killer. There are two types of inflammation namely acute inflammation and chronic inflammation.

1) Acute inflammation
Begins swiftly and becomes severe rapidly. Shows Signs and symptoms only for a few days but in some cases may continue for a few weeks.
Examples of diseases, conditions, and conditions that can result in acute inflammation consist of: Acute bronchitis, infected ingrown toenail, sore throat due to cold, a scratch or cut on the skin, exercise (especially powerful exercise), acute dermatitis, acute appendicitis, acute tonsillitis, acute infective meningitis, acute sinusitis, etc.

2) Chronic inflammation
This is actually long time inflammation, which can last for several months to even years. It may be the outcome of:

-Failure of abolition of cause of acute inflammation

-An autoimmune response to normal healthy body cells

-A chronic irritant of low strength that continue to operate undetected.

Examples of diseases and situations with chronic inflammation in are: rheumatoid arthritis, chronic peptic ulcer, asthma, tuberculosis, chronic periodontitis, ulcerative colitis and Crohn's disease, chronic active hepatitis and chronic sinusitis, hay fever etc. Rheumatoid arthritis is actually inflammation of joints and tissues surrounding them. We are more concerned with anti-inflammation and soothing diet for rheumatoid patients in these chapters in detail.

Fatty acids in body called prostaglandins control inflammation, fever, tissue swelling, and allergies. There are three different families of prostaglandins that provide three different functions in our body:

-PGE1 helps to stop inflammation, decrease allergies, boost mucous production in the stomach, decreases blood pressure, makes nerve function better and finally also helps to encourage immune response.

- PGE2 rouses the allergy response, endorses inflammation, add to platelet aggregation (sticking of platelets where the plaques form along walls of blood vessels, resulting in the development of localized or confined blood clots, that can promote block the flow of blood in the arteries), amplifies smooth muscle contraction, and suppresses immune functioning.

- PGE3 obstructs the release of pro-inflammatory prostaglandins (PGE2), increases the "good" cholesterol (HDL cholesterol), supports immune function, decreases platelet aggregation, decreases triglycerides, and reduce inflammation.

In a nut shell, we can say that PGE1 and PGE3 as the "good" prostaglandins and PGE2 as the pro-inflammatory or "bad" prostaglandin.

C) Inflammation and Chronic diseases

According to article written by Dr. Michael Noonan in 2013, health is waning rapidly because of rapid increase in chronic diseases like type 2 diabetes, chronic pain (e.g. fibromyalgia), insomnia, obesity, Alzheimer's disease, heart disease and allergies. There are some common factors that are same for all these problems, first they are all primary lifestyle diseases and secondly they all are related to chronic inflammation.

Our bodies form chemicals that naturally role in inflammation in the way that they actually resolve inflammation and these chemicals are called resolvins. Resolvins are made from dietary fats, called Omega 3 fatty acids, and a scarcity of these essential fats is one of the mainly important imbalances in our diet nowadays. The source of Omega 3 fats, in healthy amounts is most meats, unless the animal was raised on grains, where the Omega 3 fats are mostly replaced with Omega 6s. As our diets are so rich in grains and vegetable oils, we consume more Omega 6 fats and a smaller amount Omega 3s than our ancestors comparatively. This imbalance possibly contributes to chronic inflammation, and also interferes with the remedy or healing of acute injuries.

High insulin levels are another major source of body large inflammation, which is mainly caused by intake of sugary foods, as well as a diet rich in grains. All grains can generate the insulin response but refined grains like white flour and white rice, are the more dangerous.

Inflammation has impact on a few significant health conditions like heart disease, diabetes, chronic pain and insomnia.

1) Diabetes

Combined evidences from different works suggest that chronic low grade inflammation may also play role in causing type-II diabetes. According to American Journal of Clinical Nutrition (September 2005), a diet rich in inflammation producing foods, for example   refined grains, processed meats, and sugars, amplified the risk for developing type II diabetes. Another study conducted in 2001 also noted inflammation as a risk factor for diabetes in 2001by Journal of the American Medical Association.

Type 2 diabetes patients don't produce enough insulin and their bodies cannot use the insulin sufficiently. Insulin is a hormone that is made in the pancreas by cells. Function of insulin is to control the amount of sugar in the blood.

Insulin may also have effect on body tissues which is influenced by many factors, such as obesity and the accumulation of fat around some major organs in abdomen. The fat cells make chemicals those results in inflammation.

Higher levels of inflammation had been identified by researchers in the bodies of people with type 2 diabetes. The levels of certain inflammatory chemicals called cytokines inside fat tissues are noticed higher in people with type 2 diabetes comparatively in people without diabetes. They concluded that fat causes nonstop (chronic), low levels of irregular inflammation that contributes to the disease by alters insulin's action.

As type 2 diabetes begins to develop, the body becomes less responsive to insulin and the resulting insulin resistance also results in inflammation. Blood sugar levels then move stealthily higher and higher, ultimately resulting in type II diabetes.

2) Heart disease

Heart diseases are a broad term covering several conditions such as stroke, atherosclerosis, heart attack, and high blood pressure. It has been reported in "Inflammation and coronary heart disease: an overview in a journal of Cardiology in review" that in recent years, collected data revealed that certain markers of inflammationplay an important role in the development of atherosclerosis. Specially, high levels of one systemic marker of inflammation, C-reactive protein, are related to an increased risk of cardiovascular disease. Furthermore, potentially significant relations have been established between high markers of inflammation and increased effectiveness of recognized therapies.

The factors that can be checked for heart disease are blood pressure, blood glucose level, cholesterol levels, lipoprotein A, ferritin, fibrinogen, and several other factors.

Other factors involve in heart diseases are a genetic factor which means family history of heart disease, inactive and unhealthy lifestyle, smoking, infection, ischemia, damage by free radicals, inflammation, and insulin resistance.

Recent investigations have indicated that inflammation has a prominent role in the development of atherosclerotic disease.
P. Ridker in "Fibrinolytic and inflammatory markers for arterial occlusion: the evolving epidemiology of thrombosis and

hemostasis", identified inflammatory markers that make it somewhat easy to predict MI and stroke.

Another researcher A.Maseri and his coworkers examined numerous acute phase inflammatory proteins, cytokines, and intercellular adhesion molecules as prospective indicators of primary atherosclerosis and risk factor of proceeding cardiovascular events.

Risk factors or causative agents of heart diseases first stimulate the discharge of various inflammatory promoters (ROS) reactive oxygen species which are free radicals, nitric oxide , immune cells as a result of tissue injury, which results in an inflammatory reaction of the immune system as a result extended inflammation puts people at high risk for heart disease. Risk factors increase inflammation and this inflammation adds to risk for heart disease.

Types of cells those are susceptible to Cardiovascular Risk factors:

There are three types of cell that are more at risk of cardiovascular risk factors. These are:

-Epithelial cells

- Smooth muscle cells

- Immune cells.

Epithelial cells

 Line the blood vessels and have role in controlling the movement of nutrients, hormones, and immune mediators from one cell to other.

Smooth muscle cells

 Assist in controlling constriction and dilation of blood vessels which is called as vasoconstriction and vasodilation, so they are chief regulators of blood pressure.

Immune cells

Defend and repair the vascular tissue damaged from chemical and biological agents. Any disturbance to the homeostasis (balance) of these cells can lead to heart disease risk. According to an article of March 2004 in the journal name "Alternative Medicine Review", chronic inflammation is the most common damage to these three tissue types, resulting in disturbance of functioning of the cardiovascular system that is low then optimal.

Inflammation results from tissue injury or exposure to toxic chemicals cause the epithelial cells to produce a variety of molecules that add to heart disease risk. These consist of clotting and coagulation factors, fibrinolysis factors that promote abnormal bleeding, prostaglandins, nitric oxide (Vascular tone regulator)

Nitric oxide (NO) is important to mention because it plays a chief part in regulation of blood pressure because it has vasodilation promoting capabilities. In diabetes, concentration of NO will decrease, which will cause increased vasoconstriction and hypertension (increased blood pressure)

During hypertension, some smooth muscle cells, which are of elastic nature, change to more secretory cells. Smooth muscle cells are usually elastic in nature because of adaptation to the changeable blood pressure experienced throughout the day. When they change to secretory smooth muscle cells they release growth promoters and start to form a lesion of propagating secretary smooth muscle cells along the blood vessel. This lesion is clinically significant as it develops and promotes important cholesterol and lipid deposits that make the cell wall weak as the cells experience apoptosis (*a genetically determined process of cell self-destruction that is marked by the fragmentation of nuclear DNA, is activated either by the presence of a stimulus or by the removal of a stimulus or suppressing agent, is a normal physiological process eliminating DNA-damaged, superfluous, or unwanted cells (as immune cells targeted against the self in the development of self-tolerance or larval cells in amphibians undergoing metamorphosis), and when halted (as by genetic mutation) may result in uncontrolled cell growth and tumor formation—called also programmed cell death.* Merriam Webster Medical Dictionary). As this area of cells deteriorate the vascular wall, and becomes an aneurysm. An aneurysm is a clinically noteworthy cardiovascular risk factor because it has the prospective to rupture and cause immediate death.

In circumstances linked with oxidative stress that is damage to tissues by free radicals, such as high cholesterol, NO may be high but immobile, and therefore unable to promote vasodilation of blood vessels to reduce blood pressure and resist the likelihood of Aneurysm (confined blood filled balloon like swelling in the wall of a blood vessel). Inflammatory mediators in the body can be reduced through diet and reducing blood pressure through exercise and diet can also prevent us from many cardiovascular risks. So by reducing inflammation minor tissue damage can be reduced that further promotes health and prevents complications.

Mechanisms of How does the ant inflammation diet bring about all these positive changes, will be discussed latter in section of "Anti-inflammatory diet"

3) Stress and inflammation

Stress and negative emotions are every day happenings that have not only psychological inferences, but also apparent endocrine and immune consequences. These affective responses give a path by which the external environment can affects the individual's bodily processes. In addition, some evidences suggest a bidirectional association between emotions and physiological systems, in such a way that endocrine and immune changes may also change emotional responses. This is may be a special interest for social neuroscience that inflammation, which is a constituent of immune function, may be a key physiological mediator of the impact of stress and negative emotions on health.

Hundreds of years ago, humans required rapid rise in adrenaline to help them run from the tiger they came across in the forests. But the stress now we deal with occurs from stressors such as work, studies, family, traffic, buildup of toxins, and environmental stress. In stressful events, the sympathetic nervous system is activated, triggering production of a stress hormone called cortisol, which increase blood sugar to supply energy to muscle cells to run from the tiger. But if stress situations are different from that of stress of tiger then increased cortisol and blood sugar without the powerful effort of energy that is needed to run from the tiger, will cause the elevated amount of cortisol and high blood sugar level that our body does not need. In such stressful situations, many people live with continuous state of sympathetic stimulation, resulting in chronically high cortisol levels. Extended elevated cortisol can lead to blood sugar abnormalities, high blood pressure, thyroid dysfunction, increased weight, osteoporosis, hyperinsulinemia, hypercholesterolemia, and many other metabolic imbalances may occur.

Mechanism

When we came across to any psychological stress or certain physical stressors, an inflammatory process occurs by one of the following actions:

-Activation of mast cells or other inflammatory cells

- Releasing inflammatory mediators (from sensory nerves)

- Releasing neuropeptides (particularly Substance P (SP)

Neuropeptides has an action like neurotransmitters, mainly corticosteroid releasing factor (CRF), and Substance P, trigger a stress response by activating neuro-endocrinological pathway through sympathetic nervous system, , renin angiotensin system (hormone system that regulate balance of water and blood pressure)hypothalamic pituitary pathway, release stress hormones in blood. For example catecholamines (dopamine, epinephrine and nor epinephrine), corticosteroids (corticosterone, cortisol and aldosterone), growth hormone, glucagon, and renin.

These hormones in combination with cytokines provoked by stress, initiate the acute phase response (APR) and then induce the acute phase proteins which are important mediators of inflammation. Norepinephrine alone may also cause the induction of APR by macrophage activation and cytokine discharge.

Another possible factor of macrophage activation postulated by Black PH in "Stress and the inflammatory response: a review of neurogenic inflammation" is the increase in lipids with stress as many lipopolysaccharide which induces cytokines from Kupffer cells of liver, following to an increased absorption from the gastrointestinal tract during psychological stress.

The brain may start or inhibit the inflammatory process. The inflammatory response is actually present within the psychological stress response. Furthermore, the same neuropeptides that is CRF and may be SP mediate both stress and inflammation. Cytokines induced by one of this response may signal the brain by using similar somatosensory pathways.

Other occasion where stress may induce inflammatory alterations are also analyzed in the same paper that frequent episodes of acute or chronic psychogenic stress may bring chronic inflammatory changes which may result in atherosclerosis in the arteries as well as chronic inflammatory changes in other organs.

Chapter 8: Modern Health Paradigms

"New opinions are always suspected, and usually opposed, without any other reason but because they are not already common." -- (John Locke).

The main conversation in worldwide is about healthcare. This conversation is represents that how modernism in healthcare is going to be approached. Luckily, in the sphere of health care innovation, there are many people in the world, doing actual work, emerging novel ways of delivering care, and giving time, energy, liveliness and creativeness to make healthcare better.

There has been a large increase in non-communicable diseases within the last several years, and that number is still mounting. According to the Centers for Disease Control and Prevention (CDC), seven out of every ten deaths are credited to chronic diseases such as cancer, diabetes, and cardiovascular disease (heart attack and stroke etc.), all of which have a direct nutritional involvement.

The tactic for improving excellence in healthcare has progressed very fast over the past decade. This has come about because of numerous factors:

The large number of field experiences that have taken place in many countries globally and in diverse areas of expertise in healthcare delivery, lead to efficient and cost effective care. These experiences have also increased the expectations of patrons.Finally, the advances and improvement in understanding, knowledge, management, and clinical practices can also attributed to these.

At present there are at least two paradigms of healing that subsist in society.

- First paradigm, which covers diagnosis, identification and treating disease, takes a laboratory approach to ailment or

58

disorder in which the pharmaceuticals and/or surgery of patient's is done to combat symptoms. According to this approach patient is cured by curing symptoms by the use of painkillers, antibiotics, steroids, or other oppressive treatments.

- A second paradigm, holds by naturopathic medicine, examines the person entirely and acts to stimulate his or her healing, even before appearance of disease. Prevention is the keystone, in this paradigm.When someone allows the body to function properly in optimum conditions, maintains homeostasis inside the body, he/she encouragesbetter health.

Disease symptoms actually spring up to tell us that abnormal conditions or imbalance (of anything) has occurred inside the body.It directs the physician to treat these abnormalities to restore the normal good health. Symptoms sometimes appear instantly, but usually they start to develop under the surface. This paradigm move toward symptoms as indicators of something going on deeper in the body is key to finding and treating the cause of disease rather to cure only symptoms. And not just suppress them.

A) The Role of Primary Care

Primary health care within health systems is important in improving the recognition of health requirements and unfairness in summiting these needs.

Primary care is actually care given by physicians particularly qualified for and expert in inclusive first call and continuing care for persons with any unidentified signs, symptoms, or health concern not restricted by predicament origin like behavioral, biological or social, diagnosis or organ system.

The definitive objective of primary health care is better health for everyone. WHO (World Health Organization) has recognized five key fundamentals to attain that objective:

- Universal coverage reform (reducing prohibiting and social discrepancies in health)

- Service delivery reform (organizing health services about people's requirements and hopes)

- Public policy reform (incorporating health into all divisions)

- Leadership reform (following joint models of policy discussion), and

- Escalating stakeholder contribution.

According to an article published in Family Practicein 2000, many primary care doctors are hesitant to instruct patients due to their incredulity that dietary involvement can be a valuable modality, in spite of the fact that several studies have done which shows that positive dietary effects on health results. For example, Journal of the American Medical Association published a controlled test in July 2003, according to which addition of soy protein, gummy fiber, and nuts can be as useful for decreasing cholesterol as prescription statin medication to a little saturated fat diet.

 In another article published in the New England Journal of Medicine in 2002,it is stated that both diet and exercise may be more effective than pharmacologic remedy at protecting against cardiovascular diseases in patients with mess up glucose tolerance. Study on number of patients were done which showed patients had decreased their threat of developing diabetes by 58 percent after three years of diet and lifestyle changes, But when participants who were only taking metformin, which is a general pharmaceutical prescription for diabetics, decreased their diabetes risk by only 31 percent. This is a major difference.

Moreover, significant decline in C-reactive protein (CRP) in participants have also been found, which is an indirect marker of subclinical inflammation (that can't be detected through the usual diagnostic procedures) because of changes in lifestyles so it means that diseases can be controlled by changing diet.

B) Naturopathic Medicine

According to article "Naturopathy and the Primary Care Practice", published in *Journal of Family Practice*, Naturopathic medicine is a distinct type of primary care remedy that combine old age traditional healing processes with scientific advances and modern research. It is directed by a unique set of principles that make out the innate healing capacity of body, highlight disease prevention, and support person duty to get optimal health. The naturopathic physician (ND) struggles to understand each patient's state carefully in detail. Treatments address the patient's primary condition leading to disease, rather than appearing symptoms.

Naturopathy can be traced back to the European "natural cure," experienced in the nineteenth-century, when system for treating disease with natural processes such as with water, fresh air, diet, and herbs were utilized. In the beginning of 20th century, naturopathy progressed in the U.S. and Canada, by merging nature cure, homeopathy, spinal treatment and other remedies.

Naturopathic physicians use several treatment modalities. Such as:

- Nutrition analysis together with dietary for example eating more unprocessed food and using vitamins, minerals, and other supplements,
- Herbal medicines,
- Exercise therapy,
- Lifestyle analysis,
- Homeopathy,
- Hydrotherapy,
- Physiotherapy and medicines, such as therapeutic massage and joint treatment.

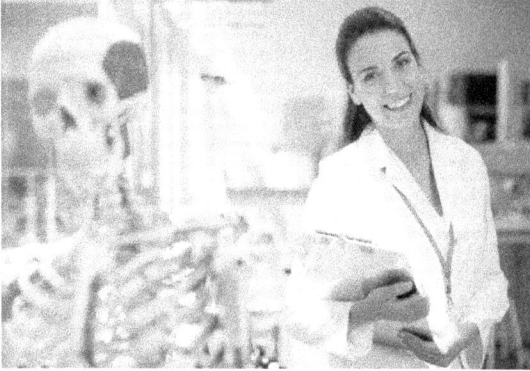

The naturopathic approach to health and disease has main focus on the restitution of health where it has get worse, the optimization of health which is necessary for good health, and the avoidance of health decline. Basically naturopathy is a mixture of traditional practices with the involvement of fresh air, fresh water, sufficient rest, nutritious and healthy food and the use of herbal therapy and nutrition to aid with the body's self-healing processes.

Various acute and chronic diseases have treated successfully with naturopathic medicines. It is beneficial in situations of treating chronic illness when allopathic medicine has failed and causing harm to body. In acute conditions, it frequently helps in the natural healing mechanism within the body. A few common conditions treated by naturopathic medicine are, allergic reactions, asthma, anxiety, depression, fatigue or weariness, digestive problems, skin problems, autoimmune diseases, thyroid illness, irregularities in menstrual, acute colds, chronic infections, and even cancer.

The underlying principles of naturopathy that help so many individuals achieve optimal health are listed below:

The healing power of nature

Naturopathic medicine recognizes the natural healing capability of body, and belief that the body has the inborn insight and intelligence to repair itself but proper direction and tools are needed.

Recognize and treat the causes

Naturopathic medicines try to recognize and treat the basic cause of disease, rather than curing appearing symptoms.

First do no harm

Begin with least involvement and continue to higher level interventions only as determined essential.

Doctor as teacher

Naturopathic doctors instruct patients, engage them in the healing course, and stress on the significance of the doctor patient affiliation.

Always treat the person entirely

Naturopathic medicine works for all features of person's health including, mental, physical, genetic, emotional, social, environmental and spiritual factors.

Give emphasis to prevention

Naturopathic medicine highlights optimal conditions and the prevention of disease

C) How Disease set on

Body will remain healthy when homeostatic system of body will be normal. Any change in this state of equilibrium or in this homeostasis makes the body susceptible to different diseases. Several physiological and psychological factors influence the balance within the body and increase the body vulnerability to diastase to.

Henry Lindlahr, M.D., in book "Philosophy of Natural Therapeutics," mentioned that one of the basic causes of disease is an unusual or abnormal composition of blood and lymph. These both are responsible for carrying nutrients to the tissues, to perform their functions, and then for bringing back wastes, toxins, and metabolic by products to the excretory sites to eliminate from the body. The composition of these fluids exclusively depend on lifestyle performances we follow and type of nutrients we take into the body through diet to give energy for very important body processes. So it means that diseases are mostly the consequence of nutrient taken less than adequate amounts so body there will be less fuel for cell metabolism.

According to another researcher Lindlahr, excess of low quality proteins, carbohydrates, and fats, in diet will cause the tissues to be blocked with "morbid matter." Thus accumulation of this toxin, can affect the vital cellular functions, so becoming pathogenic to numerous systems in the body. As a result this will cause cellular degeneration, taking the system toward disease, rather than sustaining the cellular regeneration which is required for repair and healing.

Depending on the formation and structure of the person, immune system and ability to remove accumulated wastes, diseases can be visible in various forms such as skin irritation, rashes, allergies and asthma, while one who is feeble and is less efficient at removing wastes, may accumulate waste products in the form of cysts, growths, and finally this can lead to cancer. So the body can function properly if it is balanced and is functioning optimally.

1) Germ Theory of Diseases

Louis Pasteur made the most important intellectual jump in the history of medicine, following a similarity between fermentation and disease. He realized that just as yeast and bacteria carry out fermentation, so microorganisms also cause diseases.

The *germ theory of disease* states that a number of diseases are caused by microorganisms. These organisms are very small and cannot be seen with naked eye, attack humans, animals, and other living hosts. They grow and reproduce in their living hosts and so cause much disease there. Germs may include viruses, bacteria, fungi, or prions. These are called pathogens, and diseases caused by them are called" infectious diseases".

Pasteur also developed the process of "pasteurization" by heating milk and wine to stop development of bacteria, but it had nothing to do with diseases of humans. Pasteur had no direct method of killing microorganism, but he revealed the way of prevention of rabies by vaccination, which had been fruitfully applied by Jenner to smallpox in the end period of eighteenth century.

Many physicians and researchers then worked on Pasture's idea and identified microbial cause of many diseases for example they identified that cause of rabies was rabies virus, anthrax by bacillus anthrax, typhoid fever by salmonella Typhi, tuberculosis by Mycobacterium tuberculosis, Diarrhea by Escherichia coli, Pneumonia by Streptococcus pneumonia, Meningitis by Neisseria meningitides, Food poisoning by Salmonella Enteritidis and Plague by Yersinia pestis etc..

2) Limitation of Germ theory

According to the article by Stewart G.T and his co-workers, infectious disease is principally caused by transmission of an organism from one host to another (Germ theory of disease) is like sweeping statement. It deals with the essential facts that without an organism infection is unworkable and that infectious organisms will definitely cause a disease but it does not explain the exceptions and variance. The germ theory ignores many other factors which are important in choosing the relationship host, germ and environment and genetic factors that lead to infection.

A naturopathic physician, Dr. Dickson Thom and Dr. Gerard Gueniot, a medical physicians, have always educated that disease is only able to affect a body if body is vulnerable to that disease. If homeostasis system of body has disturbed for any reason for example, non-hygienic and improper diet, unhealthy lifestyle habits, family history (genetic), emotional trauma, toxins present in environment , body becomes feeble, and immune system of body has also become weaker due to which body become more susceptible to infections. Disease can be prevented or predictable depending on the person's strength and environment.

Another microbiologist Dr. Rene Dubos had also the same opinion that Viruses and bacteria are not the only cause of the diseases there is something more.   Potentially pathogenic microbial agents continue to enter in human bodies most of the time but not all the time body becomes infected. They affect only when there is something wrong with equilibrium due to which infection   develop   into   disease.

Chapter 9: Importance of Diet in Rheumatoid Arthritis

Diet is a specific pattern of consumption and a balanced diet contributes to body's need of proper quantity of all nutrients without any surplus or scarcity for optimal growth and development and to maintain good health. People are interested in their diet to remain healthy, lose weight or to enhance their performance so that they can work more efficiently. Different nutritional plans have been designed according to differences and requirements by the body, so there is not a single diet that will meet the demands of every one. Not only a single food can supply all the nutrients our body needs, for that reason it is essential to eat a broad variety of different foods. But, some foods are required in large amount and more frequently than others.

Furthermore according to American Journal of Clinical Nutrition, many studies have revealed the significance of diet in combination with active lifestyle helps in the prevention and cure of many diseases like cancer, coronary heart disease, gastrointestinal diseases, birth defects and cataracts etc. so if our diet will have higher quality food, the more nutrients and energy we get from it and have low will be the chance of getting diseases.

A) Role of nutrition and diet in rheumatoid arthritis

In rheumatoid arthritis, immune reactions and inflammation target and surrounding parts causing pain swelling, pain and irregularity. It is very common disease now and according to the survey in 2010almost 49,000 deaths occurred globally because of rheumatoid arthritis. Rising research seems to point out a link between diet and inflammation. Though the precise mechanisms are still indistinct, yet some foods appear to protect against inflammation. Factors affecting nutrition and diet in rheumatoid arthritis are:

B) Metabolic effects of inflammation

Tumor necrosis factor α and interleukin 1β cause fever, efficient catabolism, muscle wasting, connective tissue deformation and anorexia related to RA Elevated levels of free radicals boost the oxidative stress on antioxidant resistance,said by Grimble in article "Nutrition and cytokine action" . High level of mineral like Copper, reduced plasma Zinc and Iron are some factors of inflammation which are not so much obvious, particularly in RA. Roubenoff et al published findings in article, abnormal homocysteine metabolism in rheumatoid arthritis, indicating unusual homocysteine metabolism in Rheumatoid arthritis.

1) Physical disability

Patient suffered from rheumatoid arthritis also experience physical disability. Abridged physical activity results in loss of bone mass. This not only depends on disease activity and drug therapy but also depends on vitamin D deficiency in situations where there is slight exposure to sunlight.

2) Malnutrition in rheumatoid arthritis

Increase in catabolism elevates resting energy spending, which results in loss of weight and wasting of body mass, chiefly when there is insufficient supply of energy and protein. This happening is known as "rheumatoid cachexi". A study was carried out by different researches identifying malnutrition in RA patient and was more common in patients with severe condition. Low dietary consumption of Copper, Magnesium, Zinc, vitamins D, E and A, pyridoxine, folate and n-3 fatty acids have been constantly mentioned by different researchers.

Dietary advices and food that is beneficial for RA sufferers will be discussed in later section.

C) Role of Diet in Mitigating the Effects of Toxic burden

In our daily life we come across many environmental toxins and several food byproducts gather in our body through diet through diet which are not as much required by the body and several pharmaceutical drugs used for remedy of different diseases. Ingestion of unnecessary chemicals through foods, like hormones, pesticides, antibiotic remains, and other compounds, demands body to work more efficiently so that these foreign substances can be digested in addition to getting nutrients from the same foodstuff.

Organs in the body responsible for metabolism and excretion of these toxic substances are liver and kidney. These organs have to be efficient in breaking and eliminating toxic compounds from the body. The efficiency with which individual's body eliminates these collective wastes decides his or her "terrain" which is defined as the body's vulnerability to disease due to its biochemical and energetic environment. So every individual has his own terrain.

Along with effect metabolic and excretory system, digestive system must also work hard to digest and break down airborne and food borne allergens. Digestion results in accumulation of waste byproducts and toxins in our body but there is a solution to this problem that is by reducing dietary toxins effectively can eliminate the remaining ones.

To understand the relation between stress, toxins, allergens, and metabolic and diet consider an example given by Jessica K. Black, N.D in book named "Anti inflammation diet and recipe book" that imagine you have a cup having eight fluid ounces. This cup represents your possible toxin and allergen ingestion. If the cup is filled with six ounces of food allergies, you can take in only two more ounces sooner than the cup overflow and you can no longer treat with the toxins. After then if you are exposed to environmental toxins, pollens, and pharmaceutical drugs, your cup cannot grip the entire intake to your system. As your cup spill over, you will experience runny nose, pain, cough, rash, fatigue, and much more symptoms. But On the other hand, if six ounces of food allergies are removed, you have greater ability in taking and processing toxins and allergens that are difficult to protect from. Just as patients very allergic to pollen and grass may not eliminate all of the grass and pollens from their lives, but better processing of grass and pollens can reduce their food allergies.

D) Food Intolerances, Food allergies and Inflammation

It is a general understanding that if we will take good food we will have good health. But sometimes this concept does not fit and even a fresh and good food can make an individual sick. Such as fresh strawberries can sometime elicit an allergic reaction, glass of milk can provoke stomach cramps; daily consuming bread can induce loss of weight and can cause fatigue. When ordinary food is causing health problems than one should consult health professional. It may be the consequence of food allergy and intolerance.

1) Food allergy

An instant or delayed immune reaction to a particular food, even small amount of intake of food is called as food allergy. The reaction can be easygoing, like a rash, itchiness, nausea, vomiting, diarrhea, abdominal cramps. But sometime reaction can be severe such as swelling of tongue, face, airway, and even it can become life threatening such as anaphylaxis. Body responds so because body's immune system is incorrectly recognizing that particular food as an unsafe substance that result in production of antibodies to attack the felonious food and releases histamine into the blood and thus symptoms of allergic reactions appear.

Common food allergens are:

- Peanuts
- Other nuts
- Milk
- Soy
- Wheat
- Fish
- Crustaceans (prawn, lobster, crab)
- Molluscs (oysters, octopus, muscles)
- Different fruits
- Food additives (salicylates, benzoates &derivatives of sulphites, mono sodium glutamate).

According to the estimation of Mayo Clinic, 6 to 8 percent of children below five year of age, and almost 3 to 4 percent of adults, have real food allergy that increase with age of sufferer.

2) Food Intolerance
Food tolerance is actually inability of body to digest specific type of food.
It does not involve the immune system. It happens due to lack of a specific enzyme required by body to digest a specific type of food.

Most common food intolerances are:

- Lactose intolerance,

- Milk intolerance,

- Food additive intolerance,

- Sulphites.

Food allergies and intolerances are diagnosed by healthcare professionals first by taking a full medical history to find out whether the symptoms are caused by food allergy to specific foods, or food intolerance, or due to other health related problems, keeping records of all food items taken by person.

In next step some healthcare professionals restrict a person to specific diet and eliminate diet, which is causing an allergic reactions and problems. For example, if person is suspected to allergic to egg, then egg is eliminated from his diet.

In next steps different tests are recommended to confirm diagnosis such as skin prick test and blood tests.

An oral food test is the last way by healthcare professionals in which he gives doses of different doses to find out the allergic foods.

E) Symptoms of food intolerance and food allergy

Symptoms of food intolerance and food allergy frequently overlap, they are:

- Stomach and bowel disturbance,

- Bloating and swelling,

- Migraines and headaches,

- Difficulty in breathing and sinusitis,

- Rashes,

- Suffocation,

- Anaphylaxis,

- Irritable bowel disease,

- Fatigue,

- Arthritis,

- Acne,

- Mouth ulcers,

- Ear infection,

- Mood changes.

1) *Relation Of food hypersensitivities to Rheumatoid arthritis*

R. S Panush, reported that specific foods intensify the symptoms of RA in some patients. Prevention from these foods has been shown to have restricted, short term benefits but no any long term benefits have been shown. Different dietary modification were carried out to have apparently better symptoms in some patients, but people with Rheumatoid arthritis may have unprompted brief remissions. As a result, it is significant to carry out double blind, sop controlled tests to differentiate diet effect from spontaneous remission.

Diet elimination (mentioned in previous section) analysis is carried out to determine food hypersensitivities in patients. Panush and his coworkers confirmed temporary betterment in the symptoms of RA with diet elimination and variation in a controlled study and the symptoms related to food sensitivities were then studied. During fasting period or in strictly restricted diet, the patient's symptoms improved considerably. On the other hand, when the milk was reintroduced into the diet, occurrence of pain, stiffness and swelling in joints were seen. Then Kjeldsen and his fellows observed that fasting may be effective in decreasing the symptoms of RA, but most of the patients relapsed to previous stage when new foods were introduced into their diet.

2) *Foods that can cause Inflammation*

Nicholas Perricone, MD, the pioneering dermatologist and nutritionist in his book on anti-inflammation eating reported that our bodies in fact depend on brief inflammation to help in fighting sudden injuries or infections. But when this inflammation turns into chronic, the immune system misguidedly attacks normal cells of the body, and so the process of healing becomes destructive.

The foods that can contribute to inflammation includes all dairy products, wheat products, potatoes, sugar, tomatoes, corn, citrus fruits, commercial eggs, pork, nuts, butter, coffee, alcoholic drinks, coffee, soda water, processed food and items containing hydrogenated oils.

For example, potatoes and tomatoes, can cause inflammation in patients of not only in rheumatoid arthritis but also in many other types of arthritis.

3) Dairy products

Similarly dairy foodstuffs are rich in fat. There is not a problem with fat because of fat soluble toxins that are stored in the fat. But genetically modified soy yield in the feed and toxins in the form of pesticide residues in feed increases the toxin amount in dairy products. As a consequence, dairy products interfere with body's immune system. Calcium which is important for body especially in growing children is thought to obtain mainly from milk can not only taken from dairy products but also from many non-dairy sources including fortified soy, oat, rice, almond, and in nut milks. Fortified milk is also a better choice.

30 percent of the calcium is absorbed by body from dairy products. Study of different articles it is concluded that an allergy to cow's milk is common among people. Milk proteins stimulate the release of pro-inflammatory cytokines in patients at risk of allergies. Furthermore due to acidic nature of milk proteins, the body tries to balance the pH in the gastrointestinal system by removing calcium from the bones. It has suggested in "Ant inflammation diet and recipe book" that eating organic dairy products is not bad as they don't have the pesticide residues,

antibiotic residues and hormones that regular dairy stuffs may contain but should not consumed daily.

Drinking a lot of water is suggested in this book in amount that a person having weight 140 pounds should drink seventy fluid ounces of water every day, which is equal to almost 9 cups but water should be filtered in order to protect our bodies from toxins like lead, aluminum, bacteria, pollutants from industries etc.

4) *Caffeinated and sugar containing beverages*

Caffeinated beverages and beverages containing sugar should also be avoided. Because of large amount of concentrated sugar in these beverages. We should always keep in mind that excess of everything is bad.

Coffee and other beverages containing caffeine are very toxic to the liver because of its harsh effect on adrenal gland and so has effect on cortisol levels. The adrenal glands, present on top of the kidneys, are responsible for performing many functions in body such as maintaining energy, production of sex hormones, balance of blood pressure and blood sugar level, and in stress response, on weight loss..

5) *Beef, eggs and pork*

Commercial beef, eggs and pork should also be avoided largely for the similar reasons that dairy is to be avoided: because of high content of toxins content and acidic nature of the animal protein. So their high consumption is harmful for body.

Pork and beef promotes inflammation as they are rich in arachidonic acid. Beef is allowed to some extent but Pork, even organic and minute amount, is prohibited because it stimulate an autoimmune reaction. Pigs have alike protein structures to that of humans so its consumption can raise the possibility of cross reactions in the immune system. Because pigs mostly live in untidy environments, eat anything around them, even their own young, so Jessica K.Black thinks that they have low quality fats. Organic eggs free of pesticide residues are although allowed, but not in very large quantity.

Elevated consumption of meat in rheumatoid arthritis may exacerbate the symptoms. This association between intake of meat and rheumatoid arthritis engages some distinctive features of meat digestion, chiefly the bile acids production by the liver in response to high meat intake. In certain conditions, bacteria reside in the digestive tract can get grip of these bile acids and convert them into inflammatory substances. Changing the diet to vegetarian direction may often is useful in reducing the symptoms of rheumatoid arthritis

6) Sugar

Excess sugar should be avoided by all individuals because it can cause abnormal reactions in body. High sugar consumption will contribute to diabetic condition and elevated cholesterol levels all of which are risk factors for heart disease.

7) Peanuts

Peanuts are common food allergens so they should also be avoided. Peanuts have aflatoxin on their exterior, which is potent carcinogenic in some individuals.

8) Corns

Corn is another allergen that must to be avoided because usually grown corn now used is genetically engineered product that may contain toxins.

Antibodies against proteins found in wheat have been identified in rheumatoid patients. So it is important to reduce consumption of wheat products in these patients. Oats can also sometime cause allergic reactions.

F) Diet's Role in Rheumatoid Arthritis

Diet can be one's friend or enemy in the fight against rheumatoid arthritis. Diet which is mostly recommended in RA includes:

1) Fish and Omega-3 Fatty Acids

The equilibrium of fatty acids in the body is important. If a body has sufficient omega-3 fatty acids, it can generate healthy cells for an efficient immune system. The body can more efficiently fight against viruses, bacteria, and other harmful foreign invaders. Right dietary choices are there to tell us what type of fats is essential to body in different condition of body. Cold water fish, like salmon, herring halibut, mackerel, cord and tuna are wealthy sources of these fats and have been shown to raise the amount of omega-3 fats in the body.

Researchers have recommended about 4-6 servings of these type of fish every week to reduce symptoms of rheumatoid arthritis significantly. It can take almost 3 months to see the beneficial effects of supplements so determination is important.

2) Vitamin D-rich Foods

One of the study published in the January 2004 in article "Arthritis and Rheumatics" suggests that consumption of foods high in vitamin D such as different type of sunflower seeds, fish, eggs, and vitamin D-fortified dairy products provides defense against getting rheumatoid arthritis more complicated.

Studies were carried out in number of women consuming the foods mostly naturally having high content of vitamin D were found to have a 27% lesser risk of Rheumatoid Arthritis. Those consuming the Vitamin D fortified food, like milk products, had a 34% lower risk of increasing Rheumatoid arthritis. Researchers considered that vitamin D is not only functioning as an effective regulator of calcium in body but may also have role in sustaining normal immune functions. It's Dairy foods containing high vitamin D content may also have proteins that are involved in food allergies, so if any sin or symptom then dairy foods should at once be stopped in the case of rheumatoid arthritis, and look for other source of vitamin D. Due to this reason organic dairy products are specifically recommended for patients with rheumatoid arthritis.

3) Antioxidants, Fruits and Vegetables

Antioxidants are of great importance in diet to scavenge free radicals present in body. These are found excessively in fruits and vegetables, mainly in bright colored groups such as oranges, mangoes, apricots, peppers,carrots, and tomatoes etc. The most familiar antioxidants are vitamins A, C and E and also carotenoids (b -β-cryptoxanthin, βb -carotene, lycopenes and luteins). Free radicals produced in body as a part of inflammation process which are very harmful and can damage cells antioxidants found in fruits and vegetables can play role in limiting the damage. They can also exert an anti-inflammatory response. Studies on synovial fluid cells and components of fluid gave confirmation for production of oxygen free radicals within inflamed rheumatoid joints. These very reactive oxygen species are expected to be concerned with joint damage according to B. Halliwell which he mentioned in his article "Oxygen radicals, nitric oxide and human inflammatory joint disease"

Antioxidants have a defensive role against tissue harm caused by oxygen free radicals. TNF-α provokes the expression of collagenase and IL-8 by a mechanism which was examined in cultured synovial fluid. This effect was then partly reserved by an antioxidant suggesting that antioxidants may have protecting effects in RA.

4) Eat Iron Rich Foods

Fatigue and weariness is a very common symptom of Rheumatoid arthritis and can become worse by anemia which can occur as a result of inflammationor because of prolong use of anti-inflammatory drugs. To cope with this condition iron rich foods

78

(leafy vegetables, lean meat, pulses, fortified breakfast cereals etc.) should be used regularly in diet. Body can absorb iron more easily then vitamin C.

5) Eat Calcium Rich Foods

Calcium is necessary in diet to make the bones strong and healthy. It is even more important in RA patients because of higher threat of developing osteoporosis, so sufficient calcium intake is essential. Good sources of calcium include milk, cheese, yogurt and some other dairy food items, green leafy vegetables and almonds etc. Calcium also needs vitamin D to assist its absorption.

6) Nutritional Supplements

A healthy diet is essential to the body and it must contain all the nutrients required by the body. If diet does not contain such essential components then multivitamin and mineral supplement fortification is needed. But only when prescribed by a doctor or suggested by a pharmacist.

Chapter 10: Individual'sAnti-inflammation diet Guidelines

An individual's diet must be nutritious andwell balanced to maintain energy supplies and for proper muscle functioning to protect thejoints. Normally the number of calories we consume every day will sustain our body weight healthy. But there is a problem of weight loss in patients with RA. Not only the weight loss commonly weight gain is also a main problem. Several factors are involved in these conditions such as taking medications like corticosteroids that increase appetitecan lead to weight gain.

Moreover, in some patients muscle loss occurs, which reduce themetabolic rate of body,body cannot burn enough calories. At last arthritis often restrictphysical activity, so no much energy is then needed to the body.

A nutritionally balanced diet consists of a diversity of foods from several food groups. Nutrition scientists worked on itand United States Department of Agriculture supported by the Department of Health and Human Services, developed the "The Food Guide Pyramid." And "Dietary Guidelines for Americans". From these sources we can take help.These are research base dietary systems. The major stress of these guidelines is on dropping fat and unhealthy foods and promoting good and healthy food choices. Theprinciples mentioned in these guides one can select better choice of food in different medical condition including Rheumatoid Arthritis.

When the human immune system attacks on joints, RA begins. This ultimately results into pain, stiffness and inflammation. The treatment for RA involves use of pain killers, anti-inflammatory medication and medication for depression of immune system. All these three remedies can cause a number of side effects. To avoid the bad effects for meditational treatment for RA, patient can turn to treat RA by using appropriate diet that can reduce disease causing factors as well as symptoms such as pain, inflammation, these all contribute to anti-inflammatory diet.

A) Building Blocks

The basic constituents of diet are carbohydrates, proteins and Fats. It is recommended that RA patient should reduce weight as the effected joints have to bear comparatively lesser weight. The basic nutrients which are above mentioned can only calorie diet. According to USDA standards a normal person daily calorie intake should include ¼ t part of protein and fats and almost ½ part include carbohydrates. A patient should take low calorie diet to lose weight or maintain it at appropriate level

Besides these basic ingredients, there is great variety of nutrients present in food. Each has a unique effect on body of human being .In case of RA treatment, Diet is most important aspect. There are a number of diets available that can be proved as blessing for RA patient. Anti-inflammatory foods have secret nutrient which is Omega 3 fatty acid. The food including fat containing fish like mackerel, herring, salmon, tuna and fish oil supplements contain omega 3fatty acid. Nuts also contain omega 3 fatty acids like almonds, peanuts and walnuts.
The inflammation is caused by free radicals in joints. The use of antioxidants in diet can cure this problem. Antioxidants can reduce RA symptoms including pain and inflammation. Vitamin and mineral selenium containing diets can provide antioxidant.

1) Proteins
The constant and optimum level of sugar level in body can be maintained by using good quality protein diet. 45 to 60 gram of protein daily intake can maintain good energy level in body throughout day. Protein diet should be free of pesticide grass eater meat sources, hormone and antibiotic free meat products. Lamb, Turkey and organic protein diets can be used.
Soy, soy sauce, fermented soy such as tofu can be good source as protein for meat lovers and vegetarians as a protein diet. Nuts,

81

seeds, and legumes are valuable protein sources. Legume containing meals can provide complete source of protein food. Eggs should be obtained from antibiotic free chickens, Poached, or half boiled or slow cooked for prevention from oxidation of the egg protein, are best modes to obtain valuable protein from the eggs.. Avocados rich in proteins can be used in morning and afternoon as a healthy snack.

2) Fats

The most important fact about fats is eating right fats for patient's health. Fats are taken in appropriate amount so that weight gain is minimized. Anti-inflammatory fats have crucial importance in RA diet plan. So, animal fat intake should be from organic sources, due to the ability of animals to stock up toxins in their fat tissue. In addition, nonorganic sources of fat may also come across to more toxins, antibiotics, hormones, and other some other compounds.

Types of fat

Two types of fats are there
Healthy fats
- Monounsaturated fats,

- Poly unsaturated fats.

Unhealthy fats
- Trans-fats,

- Saturated fats.

Monounsaturated fats

Monounsaturated fats are the most common type of fats present in oils obtained from plant source such as olive, peanut oils and canola, monounsaturated soft margarines, nuts and avocados etc. These fats help in lowering cholesterol levels in blood. Therefore it is recommended to replace saturated and Trans fats in diet with polyunsaturated or monounsaturated fats. It is also called good fat as it lowers the bad LDL cholesterol and increase good HDL cholesterol in body thereby lowering the risk of heart diseases.

Polyunsaturated fats

Polyunsaturated fats are necessary for our health. They are of two types:

- Omega-6

- Omega-3

These are called as essential fatty acids because body cannot produce these fatty acids so must be taken in diet.

Omega 3 fatty acids are found in Cold water fish such as pilchards, salmon, mackerel, and sardine. These are also present in small quantities in plant foods such as flaxseeds, rapeseed, linseed oils, soya, walnuts and flax. These fats are significant in preventing the blood from clotting,regulate the heart beat and so prevent risk of heart attack, help in brain and spinal cord function and sustain healthy immune system. Omega 3 fatty acids are also required for eye and brain development of the growing fetus during pregnancy

Omega-6 type fats are found in vegetable oils such as canola, soybean and sunflower, nuts, salad dressing, and whole wheat bread. These are vital for growth, maintaining a healthy immune system; improve insulin resistance, decrease blood pressure and Lowerlevel of cholesterol.

Saturated fatty acids are solid at room temperature. These include hard fats like butter, lard, fats in meat and meat products, pastries, in dairy products, cakes, biscuits. Our diet should not have more than one third of our total fat intake come from saturated fat. They increase LDL in our body.

Trans fatty acids are simply liquid oils that turned into solid fats while food processing. Small amount of trans-fat id found naturally in some meat and dairy products, but trans-fat that is present in processed foods is very harmful to health. It also increases LDL and decrease HDL.

Almost 65 gram fat is recommended daily.

3) Carbohydrates

Unprocessed complex carbohydrates that are close to natural state are beneficial. These are found in fruits, vegetables, breads, dairy products, sweet potatoes, lentils beans, brown rice and barley etc. These are all good and complex sources of carbohydrates. Our body makes glucose by using these sources, which is major energy source in our body. These are also source of vitamin B, and legumes taken with grains are an immense source of absolute protein.

Carbohydrates found in processed, refined and sweetened foods, should are simple carbohydrates and their use should be very low in diet. Sources of simple carbohydrates are sugars, white flour, doughnuts, pastries, cookies, caffeinated beverages, soda pop, white rice, Simple carbohydrates elevate blood sugar levels and also make the body to increase insulin production, which in turn elicits synthesis of cholesterol.

20 to 70 grams of carbohydrates are recommended daily depending on type of activities.

4) Dietary Fiber

It is not any specific nutrient, but it is vital digestive roles

Dietary fiber consists of lignin and non-digestible carbohydrates and lignin that are intact in plants. Sources of dietary fibers are vegetables, wheat and several types of grains. Foods having high content of soluble fiber consist of fruits, barley, oat and beans.

Wide research has been carried out to observe the effects of dietary fiber and it is concluded that a low intake of fiber may be linked to a number of diseases. Dietary fibers have laxative effects and these are found to have role in relief of constipation in the elderly,young and pregnant.Fibers may be helpful in weight and in the control of diseases such as diabetes and hyperlipidemia. Also assist in increasing transit time to prevent the absorption of more toxins into the bloodstream because the stool has to stay in the rectum for some time, reduce the effect of food allergies, develop the body's ability to make use of nutrients, and keep the digestive environment clean. 35 grams of fiber per day are recommended by National Institutes of Health.

B) Food that should be used to prevent inflammation

In short to decreases inflammation following foods should be used in diet:

- Cold water fish, oily fish like salmon, tuna etc. and oils extracted from fish. 2 servings per month are necessary because of presence of essential fatty acid

- Particular type of fruits (apricots, cranberries, blackberries, papayas, plums, peaches,Apples, cherries, pears, grapes, pomegranates, pineapples and figs.1 to 2 serving of any fruit per day is essential)

- Vegetables (mustard and dandelion greens, spinach, radishes,onion, turnips, red pepper, parsley pumpkin, beet,cauliflower etc.3 to 5 servings or even more of green vegetables per day should be included in diet)

- Garlic, ginger, and turmeric (natural detoxifier, antibacterial, and anti-inflammatory. Should use in cooking)

- Most important is filtered water (9 to 10 cups per day)

- Bread, rice, cereals and Pasta (Recommendation: six to eleven servings daily in RA patients)

- Milk, Cheese and yogurt (Recommendation: two to three serving)

C) Life style choices in RA
Changing physical activities, eating habits and managing stress help in feeling

1) Healthy Eating in RA Management

Adopting healthy lifestyle can help RA patient in managing the disease Although there is not a miracle type of diet but eating more fruits and vegetables mentioned in previous section and use of unsaturated fats specially in fish oils can do some work.

2) Physical exercise

Different researchers observed that exercise has a major role in managing RA. It not only makes the joint flexible to move but also helps patients in maintain a healthy weight, which can assist in lessen some of the symptoms of the disease. When people gain weight, they raise the stress positioned on their joints, so making arthritis worse in such a way.

3) Emotional Health and RA

Getting rid of depression is in fact essential in people with Rheumatoid arthritis and also in other chronic diseases. Depression has found in almost one third of patients of RA. Past studies have revealed that stress and depression cause greater sensitivity to pain. It brings the feeling of helplessness. Symptoms of stress then results in fatigue, further disturbance in immune system functioning and weight gain. All these conditions make the situation more badly.

Focusing on positive thoughts, meditation, making time for exercise and relaxation, cognitive-behavioral therapy, progressive muscle relaxation can make emotional health better.

Chapter 11: Best & Tasty Recipes for RA-Patients

A) Appetizers, Side Dishes, Seasonings, and Spreads

Appetizer Recipe #1: Healthy Asparagus in Sweet Lemon

Ingredients:

- One tablespoon ground cashews (optional-for garnish),

- Two bunch asparagus (abt. 1 pound),

- Juice of onestandard size lemon,

- Three tablespoons olive oil,

- ¼ teaspoon ground nutmeg,

- ¼ teaspoon pepper (black),

- ½ teaspoon sea salt

Options: You can add green beans in the recipe. Nutritional facts per serving for Healthy Asparagus in Sweet Lemon:

Nutrients	Value
-CALORIES	128.4
-PROTEIN	2.9 G
-CARBOHYDRATE	6.2 G
-FIBER	2.6 G
-SATURATED FAT	1.7 G
-TOTAL FAT	11.3 G
-CHOLESTEROL	0.0 MG
-SODIUM	293.7 MG

Appetizer Recipe #2: Zero Cholesterol Versatile Pesto

- Fresh and washed 4 cups fresh basil leaves,

- 1/3 cup pine nuts,

- ¼ teaspoon pepper (for taste if desired),

- ¼ teaspoon salt,

- ½ cup olive oil (extra-virgin only),

- Three to four cloves of garlic

Options: Parsley, Spinach or cilantro can be used instead of basil leaves to vary taste as per liking.

Nutritional facts per serving for Zero cholesterol Versatile Pesto:

Nutrients	Value
-CALORIES	330.6
-PROTEIN	2.7 G
-CARBOHYDRATE	4.1 G
-FIBER	2.1 G
-SATURATED FAT	4.3 G
-TOTAL FAT	35.1 G
-CHOLESTEROL	0.0 MG
-SODIUM	146.8 MG

Spreading Recipe #1: Hummus (Nut 'n' Curry)

- Three cups cooked garbanzo beans,

- ½ –1 teaspoon sea salt, or to taste,

- Paprika/parsley or both (for garnish),

- ½ cup almond butter,

- Two teaspoons curry powder,

- Lemon juice (¼ cup plus 1 tablespoon fresh),

- ¼ cup liquid from garbanzo beans,

- 1/3 cup tahini (easily available in all super-stores),

- Three garlic cloves (minced or crushed),

- Three tablespoons filtered water

Options: Mixed all ingredients together and blend them until it becomes a sauce. Pour and serve. To increase or change the taste some vegetables like carrot or reddish can also be added.

Nutritional facts per serving for Hummus (Nut 'n' Curry):

Nutrients	Value
-CALORIES	356
-PROTEIN	13 G
-CARBOHYDRATE	31.9 G
-FIBER	8.0 G
-SATURATED FAT	2.4 G
-TOTAL FAT	21.9 G
-CHOLESTEROL	0.0 MG
-SODIUM	300.9 MG

B) Breads

Bread Recipe #1: Delicious Rice-Flour Bread

Ingredients:

- Three eggs (gently beaten),

- Two cups tapioca flour,

- 1¼ cups soy milk,

- Two cups rice flour,

- ½ cup warm water,

- One teaspoon vinegar,

- Four tablespoons melted organic butter,

- 1½ teaspoons sea salt,

- Four teaspoons xanthan gum (easily available in all major food stores),

- Four teaspoons dry yeast granules,

- Two teaspoons plus ¼ cup honey

Options: Coconut oil and different flours can be added in the recipe to add flavor and vary nutrition.

Nutritional facts per serving for Delicious Rice-Flour Bread:

Nutrients	Value
-CALORIES	533.9
-PROTEIN	10.2 G
-CARBOHYDRATE	96.7 G
-FIBER	3.5 G
-SATURATED FAT	6.0 G
-TOTAL FAT	12.1 G
-CHOLESTEROL	126.3 MG
-SODIUM	740.1 MG

C) Breakfasts

Breakfast Recipe #1: "Quick & Easy 5 Minute Breakfast":

Ingredients:

- ¼ cup walnuts (chopped),

- Optional - ½ teaspoon maple syrup,

- One cup brown rice (leftover cooked),

- ¼ cup sunflower (seeds),

- ¼ teaspoon cinnamon powder,

- ½ cup rice milk/ any other milk,

- 1/8 cup raisins,

- Optional - ¼ teaspoon carob powder

Options: You can change or add any seeds or nuts to bring flavor and variations to this recipe.

Nutritional facts per serving for Quick & Easy 5 Minute Breakfast:

Nutrients	Value
-CALORIES	370.5
-PROTEIN	11.0 G
-CARBOHYDRATE	40.7 G
-FIBER	5.2 G
-SATURATED FAT	2.2 G
-TOTAL FAT	20.4 G
-CHOLESTEROL	0.0 MG
-SODIUM	28.2 MG

D) Teas & Beverages

Tea Recipe #1: "Mind Relaxing Tea":

Ingredients:

- Two(parts) peppermint,

- One(part) hibiscus flowers,

- One(part) catnip,

- One(part) basil,

- One(part) lemon balm.

Tea Recipe #2: "Stomach Friendly Tea":

Ingredients:

- Two(parts) peppermint,

- One(part)fennel,

- One(part)anise seed,

- Oneand a half (part)gingerroot.

Tea Recipe #3: "Immune System- booster rocket Tea":

Ingredients:

- Two(parts) elderberry,

- Two(parts)echinacea,

- One(part)hyssop,

- One(part)thyme,

- One(part)licorice,

- Two(parts) peppermint.

Tea Recipe #4: "Wonderful Sleep Tea":

Ingredients:

- Two(parts) chamomile,

- One(part)passion-flower,

- Optional-One(part)valerian,

- Two(parts) skullcap.

Beverages Recipe #1: "Tasty Almond Milk":

- One cup whole almonds (raw),

- Three cups filtered water (amount can be varied according to taste and liquefaction desired). Blend the raw almonds in desired amount of water and get yourself a tasty and equally healthy almond milk shake. Remember to soak the almonds in the water overnight to extract their milk in the recipe.

E) Grains

Grains recipe #1: "Healthy Oats":

Ingredients:

- One cup oats

- Two cups fresh water

Options: You can add fruits and vegetables for taste.

F) Salads

Salad recipe #1: "Beans & Avocado Salad":

Ingredients for salad:

- Twomedium size ripe avocados (cut into small cubes),

- Three cups beans (black, kidney, green, pinto). Use cooked and tries to add at least three different kinds of beans.

- ½ cup green pepper (chopped in small cubes),

- ½ cup red pepper (chopped in small cubes),

- Six large lettuce leaves.

Ingredients for dressing on the salad:

- Olive oil,

- Rice vinegar,

- Raw honey,

- Fresh parsley,

- Fresh coriander leaves, - ½ teaspoon black pepper

Options: You can add both vegetables and fruits to your salad but keeping it original will bring more taste and health.

Nutritional facts per serving for Beans & Avocado Salad:

Nutrients	Value
-CALORIES	476.9
-PROTEIN	9.2 G
-CARBOHYDRATE	37.5 G
-FIBER	12.1 G
-SATURATED FAT	4.7 G
-TOTAL FAT	34.1 G
-CHOLESTEROL	0.0 MG
-SODIUM	8.3 MG

Chapter 12: Coping with the Pain & Joint Protection in Rheumatoid Arthritis

A) Protect Your Joints

Joints and muscles should be in perfect condition in order to spend a normal-healthy life. Slightest of pain or discomfort in the body can disturb the whole lifestyle. Every day jobs become more difficult and sometimes lead to frustration. If you are a rheumatoid arthritis patient yourself, you must already be practicing something to protect your joints from pain. While doing so, you might not be having a pleasant experience but surely you will reap the benefits in long term. There are so many options available these days to both protect your joints and reduce stiffness, inflammation and pain in joints. Always try to add things to your daily life so that more and more additions (exercise, diet, therapies & gadgets) will take you in a proper comfort zone. For professionals mostly involved in physical activities, using protective methods, handful tools and therapies will definitely result in less pain and fatigue.

B) Why we need to protect our joints?

Wrong living habits can cause serious damage and pain to our body. It is very common element in most of the patients, as they stand, sit and move wrongly in daily routine. Incorrect standing or sitting positions can result in great pain, especially in neck and back. For example, a slouched posture will raise stain on your neck and back. Similarly, sitting in an inappropriate position for a longer duration will also increase pain and stiffness in joints. Nonetheless, lifting heavy weights or exerting extra force in any action can also increase body strain.

Most of the people have this habit to develop specific physical movements that may not seem harmful in normal routine. However, for rheumatoid arthritis patients they can cause fatigue and additional pain. It is also very important that we find better ways to perform our daily life activities, ensuring protection of our joints and less fatigue by doing things differently. Always try to bring small changes with one change at a time to ensure it becomes a habit. Use step by step techniques to do things differently like lifting weights. You can drag things in order to move them rather picking them up to do so. Dragging will do better for you. There are countless similar examples available. Just observe what things that require change in your daily routine and try to accomplish all modifications one by one.

C) Changing your habits

Please remember that some patients might not experience any benefits by doing things differently, but one focus should be on time saving. It is obvious that both medical treatments and complementary therapies can consume lot of valuable time. Saving time by doing some tasks easily and quickly will allow you to spend more time in doing targeted exercises. So, sooner you change your habits, the better for you to control your agony. Rheumatoid and other forms of arthritis may cause deformation to some joints over a prolonged period. For instance, if a patient is suffering from rheumatoid arthritis, he can experience a deformation in wrist joints where wrist starts to point downwards. Also, the fingers can point away from the thumb at the same time. In this kind of situation, a patient should to be conscious while doing activities like opening a can, lifting a heavy item or doing any activity that can put hard pressure on the ends of the thumbsand fingers. Gripping should also be gentler to minimize any potential harm to joints. If you or any of your known individual is a rheumatoid arthritis patient and is experiencing such things, please implement some basic changes in your life to improve your situation.

D) Basic Principles to protect your joints

Some basic principles that you should practice and make a habit of them are:

- Always make sure to use your larger and stronger muscles to do most of your activities. For example, place a bag on your shoulders rather than carrying it with the hands.

- Minimize your effort and reduce stress on the joints. Use assistive devices and labor saving equipment.

- Avoid anything that has to do with twisting hands, fingers and feet.

- Avoid loading pressure/force on any one of your joints alone. Try to distribute pressure to multiple joints to reduce its effect.

- Keep changing your position if you need to sit or stand at particular place for a longer duration.

- Perform all your activities smoothly in a rhythmic action. Do not haste while performing any physical activity.

Useful Practical Tips:

1. Take Proper Breaks: Train yourself to take small, regular breaks from whatever you are doing.

2. Every 5–10 minutes, Stretch the joints & muscles you are using for 30–60 seconds.

3. Try to move around every 15–30 minutes or so.

4. Set up an alarm on your computer, kitchen timer, or cell phone to remind yourself to take micro-breaks.

1) *Right Posture

The natural balance of the human body is a true miracle of nature and is ideal to perform unlimited tasks easily. Regardless of the nature of physical work, our body possesses the ability to multiply strain to different parts of the body keeping it save from potential damage of higher intensity. All these things can be said for normal people but the situation is rather complicated for rheumatoid arthritis patients. As these patients have to maintain right postures because their musculoskeletal system is no longer normal like other human beings. A right posture, enabling better alignment will ensure that the balance of the whole body is maintained accurately.

a) *Standing Posture*: The right way to keep your standing posture accurate is to align your shoulder and ears (Place in a line or arrange so as to be parallel or straight). Don't be too rigid in your posture while standing but enough to keep the hips, ankles and knees are three in line. This way, your whole body weight will be distributed equally.

b) *Sitting Posture*: First of all, make sure that you don't use any chair with a seat that is too low. The right height of a seat is where both your legs are placed on the floor in a 90 degree angle. Similarly place your back on to the chair and keep it as straight as possible and avoid bending your back for extended duration. It is very important to make small movements while sitting, because such movements will provide flexibility in your body. This flexibility will protect you from having back and neck pain. In addition to your sitting postures, also use good quality and technically engineered furniture. Low quality furniture can put extra strain on your joints and muscles.

 c) *Walking & Running*: Always make sure to but best quality pair of shoes for walking and running. Running or walking the right way is equally important for rheumatoid arthritis patients to ensure protection of the joints from pain and any potential damage. Make a habit of looking forward with your heat straight while walking or running. Looking downwards or lean shape can increase pressure on joints and exhaust your energy.

d) *Lifting & moving*: If you are required to a job that involves lifting and dragging heavy objects then make sure that you are properly trained by your employers to perform such jobs safely. Appropriate training will guide you to perform your duties safely without harming yourself. However, it is better to avoid such jobs if you are experiencing joint or muscle pain, or if you are an arthritis patient already.

Practical Tips for daily life:

- Your chair or sofa should have a firm seat

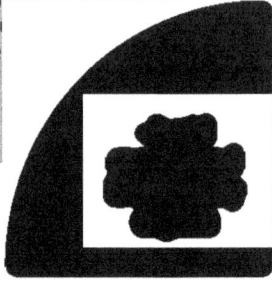

- Put a board/cushion under a saggy seat or sofa

- Sit with your hips and knees are at straight angles

- Ensure to have a supportive back rest

100

Chapter 13: Medical Treatment for Rheumatoid Arthritis

Rheumatoid arthritis is a less common type of arthritis as compared to other types like osteoarthritis. Although, it mainly involves joints and tendons in the body but other parts like heart, eyes, lungs, blood vessels and skin can also be effected with increase in severity. Pharmaceutical industry has developed specific and immensely potent medications for treatment of rheumatoid arthritis. Symptoms and pain related to rheumatoid arthritis can be effectively controlled, if the treatment gets started within the first six months of the disorder onset. Following are some commonly prescribed medications for rheumatoid arthritis.

1) HYDROXYCHLOROQUINE

Drug's most popular indications are:

- Rheumatoid arthritis

- Malaria

- SLE

- Sjögren's Syndrome

- Porphyria cutaneatarda

- Malaria Prophylaxis.

Drug's most commonly knownside effects are:

Common side-effects:

- Nausea

- Vomiting

- Headache

- Dizziness

- Irritability

- Muscle weakness

- Bleaching of hair

- Alopecia

- Pruritus

- Skin & musculoskeletal pigmentation changes

- Weight loss, anorexia

Serious side-effects:

- Blurred vision

- Photophobia

- Aplastic anemia

- Leukopenia

- Thrombocytopenia

- Cardiomyopathy (rare)

- Retinal damage with long-term use

- Corneal changes or deposits

- Visual disturbances

Recommended Dose for rheumatoid arthritis patients is:400-600 mg (310-465 mg base) PO daily for 4-12 weeks. The maintenance dose to follow is: 200-400 mg (155-310 mg base) PO daily.

2) AZATHIOPRINE

Drug's most popular indications are:

- For the prophylaxis of transplant rejection in patients receiving allogenic kidney, liver, heart.

- In immunosuppressive regimens as an adjunct to immunosuppressive agents.

Drug's most commonly knownside effects are:

- Skin rashes

- Alopecia

- Fever

- Arthralgias

- Diarrhea

- Steatorrhea

- Negative nitrogen balance

- Reversible interstitial pneumonitis

- Hepatosplenic T-cell lymphoma

- Sweet's Syndrome.

Dose limitations & recommendations for rheumatoid arthritis patients: 0.5mg/kg-2.5mg/kg per day.

Most popular brands available in the market are AZARIN, AZATHIOPRINE, and IMURAN.

3) METHOTREXATE

Drug's most popular indications are:

- Rheumatoid arthritis

- Juvenile rheumatoid arthritis

- Status epilepticus

- Seizures in neurosurgery

- Adjunct in epilepsy

- Bone marrow transplantation

- Breast cancer

- Choriocarcinoma

- Endometriosis

- Gastric cancer

- Graft rejection

- Leukaemia

- Mycoses

- Non-hodgkin's lymphoma

- Osteosarcoma

- Ovarian cancer

- Pityriasis

- Premedication

- Psoriasis

- Crohn's disease

- Systemic lupus erythematosus

Drug's most commonly known side effects are:

- Ocular irritation

- Desquamation

- Pneumonitis

- Vasculitis

- Pleuritis

- Nausea

- Vomiting

- Fever

- Erythema

- Cough

- Coma

- Seizures

- Eelvated hepatic enzymes

- Chemical arachnoiditis

- Motor paralysis of extremities

- Cranial nerve palsy

- Dementia

- Nuchal rigidity

- Myelosuppression

- Nephrotoxicity

- GI mucositis

Dose limitations & recommendations for rheumatoid arthritis patients: 7.5 mg orally weekly.

Most popular brands available in the market are EMTHEXATE PF, METHOTREXATE, UNITREXATE and METHOCIP.

4) PENICILLAMINE

Drug's most popular indications are:

- Rheumatoid arthritis

- Lead poisoning

- Arsenic poisoning

- Cystinuria

- Wilson's disease

- Chronic active hepatitis

Drug's most commonly known side effects are:

Common side effects:

- Diarrhea

- Nausea

- Anorexia

- Dysgeusia

- Anorexia

- Vomiting

Serious side effects:

- Tinnitus

- Goodpasture's syndrome

- Renal failure

- Proteinuria

- Bone marrow suppression

- Pemphigus

- Optic neuritis

Dose limitations & recommendations for rheumatoid arthritis patients: 125-250mg/day.

Most popular brand available for this generic in the market is REMINYL.

5) LEFLUNOMIDE

Drug's most popular indications are:

- Rheumatoid arthritis

- Psoriatic arthritis

Drug's most commonly known side effects are:

- Hair loss

- Indigestion

- Weight loss

- Weakness

- Bronchitis

- Pale skin

- Pale stools

- Dark urine

- Runny rose

- Back pain

- Diarrhea

- Allergic reactions

- Rash

- Hives

- Itching

- Blisters

- Burning

- Numbness

- Tingling

- Chest pain

Dose limitations & recommendations at start for rheumatoid arthritis patients: 100mg once daily for 3 days.

Most popular brands available for this generic in the market are APETOID, ARTHFREE, LEFLUMINE, AVARA, RAFIX and VAMID.

6) ABATACEPT

Drug's most popular indications are:

- Adult Rheumatoid Arthritis (RA)

- Juvenile Idiopathic Arthritis

Drug's most commonly known side effects are:

- Diarrhea

- Cough

- Fever

- Abdominal pain

- Hypertension

- Infection

- Immunizations

- Immunosuppression

Dose limitations & recommendations at start for adult rheumatoid arthritis patients:

- Body weight <60kg, 500mg with # of vials 2; Body weight 60 – 100kg, 750mg with # of vials 3;

- Body weight >100kg, 1000mg with # of vials 4, and for Juvenile Idiopathic Arthritis the recommended dosing is: - Pediatric patient <75 kg receives 10mg/kg;

- Pediatric patient weighing more than>75 kg receives no more than 1000mg.

Most popular brand available for this generic is ORENCI

References

- *Living with Rheumatoid Arthritis*, by Tammi L. Shlotzhauer. Johns Hopkins University Press, 2014.

- *Rheumatoid Arthritis,* by Marc C. Hochberg, Alan J. Silman, Josef S. Smolen, Michael E. Weinblatt, Michael H. Weisman.

* Lawrence RC, Helmick CG, Arnett FC et al. Estimates of the prevalence of arthritis and selected musculoskeletal disorders in the United States. Arthritis Rheum 1998; 41:778– 99.

* Yelin E and Callahan LF. The economic cost and social and psychological impact of musculoskeletal conditions. Arthritis Rheum 1995; 38:1351– 1362.

* Wyke B. The neurology of joints: a review of general prinicples. Clin Rheum Dis 1981; 7:223– 239.

* Schaible HG and Grubb BD. Afferent and spinal mechanisms of joint pain. Pain 1993; 55:5– 54.

* Melzack R, Wall PD: Pain mechanisms: A new theory. Science. 150:971– 979, 1965.

* Dexter D, Brandt K. Distribution and predictors of depressive symptoms in osteoarthritis. J Rheumatol 1993; 21:279– 286.

* Davis MA, Ettinger WH, Neuhaus JM, Barclay JD, Segal MR. Correlates of knee pain among U.S. adults with and without radiographic knee osteoarthritis. J Rheumatol 1992; 19(12): 1943– 1948.

* Wegener ST. Psychosocial aspects of rheumatic disease: The developing biopsychosocial framework. Curr Opin Rheumatol 1991; 3:300– 304.

* Summers MN, Haley WE, Reveille JD, Alarcon GS. Radiographic assessment and psychologic variables as predictors of pain and functional impairment in osteoarthritis of the knee or hip. Arthritis Rheum 1988; 31:204– 209.

* Lorig K, Chastain, RL, Ung E, et al. Development and evaluation of a scale to measure perceived self-efficacy in people with arthritis. Arthritis Rheum 1989; 32:37– 44.

* Fries JF, Spitz P, Kraines RG et al. Measurement of patient outcome in arthritis. Arthritis Rheum 1980; 23:137– 145.

* Lequesne MG, Mery C, Samson M et al. Indexes of severity for osteoarthritis of the hip and knee. Scand J Rheumatol 1987; 65S:85– 89.

* Bellamy N, Buchanan WW, Goldsmith H et al. Validation study of WOMAC: A health status instrument for measuring clinically important patient relevant outcomes to antirheumatic drug therapy in patients with osteoarthritis of the hip or knee. J Rheumatol 19; 15:1833– 1840.

* Crook J, Rideout E , Browne G. The prevalence of pain complaints in a general population. Pain 1984; 18:299– 314.

* McCarthy C, Cushnaghan J, Dieppe P. Osteoarthritis. In: Wall PD, Melzack R (eds.), Textbook of Pain, 3rd edition. Edinburgh: Churchill Livingstone, 1994.

* Arnoldi CC, Djurhuus JC, Heerfordt J et al. Intraosseous phlebography, intraosseous pressure measurements and 99mTc polyphosphate scintigraphy in patients with various painful conditions in the hip and knee. Acta Orthopaedica Scandinavica 1980; 51:19– 28.

* Brandt KD and Slemenda CW. In: Schumacher HR, Klippel JH, Koopman WJ (eds.), Primer on the Rheumatic Diseases, 10th edition. Atlanta: The Arthritis Foundation, 1993.

* American College of Rheumatology Ad Hoc Committee on Clinical Guidelines. Guidelines for the initial evaluation of the adult patient with acute musculoskeletal symptoms. Arthritis Rheum 1996; 39:1– 8

* Williams HJ, Ward JR, Egger MJ et al. Comparison of naproxen and acetaminophen in a two-year study of treatment of osteoarthitis of the knee. Arthritis Rheum 1993; 36:1196– 1206.

* Bradley JD, Brandt KD, Katz BP et al. Comparison of an antiinflammatory dose of ibuprofen, an analgesic dose of ibuprofen, and acetaminophen in the treatment of patients with osteoarthritis of the knee. N Eng J Med 1991; 325:87– 91.

* McCormack K. Nonsteroidal antiinflammatory drugs and spinal nociceptive processing. Pain 1994; 59:9– 43.

* Fort J. Celecoxib, a COX– 2– specific inhibitor: The clinical data. Am J Orthopedics 1999; 28(3Supp):13– 18.

* Harden RN, Bruehl SP, Backonja MM. The use of opioids in treatment of chronic pain: An examination of the ongoing controversy. J Back Musculoskel Rehab 1997; 9:155– 180.

* Ytterberg SR, Maren ML, Woods SR. Codeine and oxycodone use in patients with chronic rheumatic disease pain. Arthritis Rheum 1998; 41(9):1603– 1612

* Hochberg MC, Altman RD, Brandt KD et al. Guidelines for the medical management of osteoarthritis. Arthritis Rheum 1995; 38:1535– 1546.

* Mao J, Price DD, Mayer DJ. Experimental mononeuropathy reduces the antinociceptive effects of morphine: Implications for common intracellular mechanisms involved in morphine tolerance and neuropathic pain. Pain 1995; 61:353– 364.

* Katz WA. The role of tramadol in the management of musculoskeletal pain. Today's Therapeutic Trends 1995; 13:177– 186.

* Scnitzer TJ, Kamin M, Olson WH. Tramadol allows reduction of naproxen dose among patients with naproxen-responsive osteoarthritis pain. A randomized, double-blind, placebo controlled study. Arthritis Rheum 1999:42(7):1370– 1377.

* Wollheim FA. Current pharmacologic treatment of osteoarthritis. 1996; 52Suppl3:27– 38.

* Monks R. Psychotropic drugs. In:Wall PD, Melzack R (eds.), Textbook of Pain, 3rd edition. Edinburgh: Churchill Livingtone, 1994.

* Carette S, McCain GA, Bell DA, Fam AG. Evaluation of amitriptyline in primary fibrositis : A double-blind, placebo-controlled study. Arthritis Rheum 1986; 29:655– 659.

* Deal CL, Schnitzer TJ, Lipstein E et al. Treatment of arthritis with topical capsaicin: A double-blind trial. Clin Ther 1991; 13:383– 395.

* McCarthy GM and McCarty DJ. Effect of topical capsaicin in the therapy of painful osteoarthritis of the hands. J Rheumatol 1992; 19:604– 607.

* Algozzine et al. Trolamine salicylate cream in osteoarthritis of the knee. JAMA 1982; 247:1311– 1313.

* Acupuncture. NIH Consensus Statement. 1997 Nov 3– 4; 15(5):1–

* McAlindon TE, Felson DT, Zhang Y et al. Relation of dietary intake and serum levels of vitamin D to progression of osteoarthritis of the knee among participants of the Framingham study. Ann Int Med 1996; 125:353– 359.

* McAlindon TE, Jacques P, Zhang Y et al. Do antioxidant micronutrients protect against the development and progression on knee osteoarthritis? Arth Rheum 1996:39(4); 648– 656.

* Pipitone VR. Chondroprotection with chondroitin sulfate. Drugs Exp Clin Res 1991; 17:3.

* Morreale P. Comparison of the antiinflammatory efficacy of chondroitin sulfate and diclofenac sodium in patients with knee osteoarthritis. J Rheumatol 1996; 23:1385.

* Leeb BF, Petera P, Neumann K. [Results of a multicenter study of chondroitin sulfate (Condrosulf) use in arthroses of the finger, knee and hip joints] {German}. Wiener Medizinische Wochenschrift 1996; 146:604– 614.

* Barclay TS, Tsourounis C, McCart GM. Glucosamine. Ann Pharmacother 1998; 32:574– 579.

* Drovanti A. Therapeutic activity of oral glucosamine sulfate in osteoarthritis: A placebo-controlled double-blind investigation. Clin Ther 1980; 3:260.

* Qi GX, Gao SN, Giacovelli G et al. Efficacy and safety of glucosamine sulfate versus ibuprofen in patients with knee osteoarthritis. Arzneimittelforschung 1998; 48:469– 474. Vas AL.

* Doubleblind clinical evaluation of the relative efficacy of ibuprofen and glucosamine sulfate in the management of osteoarthritis of the knee in outpatients. Curr Med Res Opin 1982; 8:145– 149.

* Creamer P. Intra-articular corticosteroid injections in osteoarthritis: do they work and if so, how? Ann Rheum Dis 1997; 56:634– 36.

* Adams ME, Atkinson MH, Lussier AJ et al. The role of viscosupplementation with hylan G– F 20 (Synvisc) in the treatment of osteoarthritis of the knee: A Canadian multicenter trial comparing hylan G– F 20 alone, hylan G– F 20 with nonsteroidal antiin-flammatory drugs (NSAIDs) and NSAIDs alone. Osteoarthritis and Cartilage 1995; 3:213– 225.

* Balazs EA and Denlinger JL. Viscosupplementation: A new concept in the treatment of osteoarthritis. J Rheumatol 1993; supp 39; 20:3– 9.

* Scale D, Wobig M, Wolpert W. Viscosupplementation of osteoarthritic knees with hylan: A treatment schedule study. Current Therapeutic Research 1994; 55:220– 232.

* Yasui T, Akatsuka M, Tobetto K. Effects of hyaluronan on the production of stromelysin and tissue inhibitor of mettaloproteinase– 1 in bovine articular chondrocytes. Biomedical Research. 1992; 13:343– 348.

* Tobetto K, Nakai K, Akatsuka M, et al: Inhibitory effects of hyaluronan on neutrophil mediated cartilage degredation. Connect Tissue Res 1993; 29:181– 190.

* Armstrong S, Read R, Ghosh P. The effects of intraarticular hyaluronan on cartilage and subchondral bone changes in an ovine model of early osteoarthritis. J Rhematol. 21:680– 688, 199.

* Brandt KD. Osteoarthritis. In: Harrison's Principles of Internal Medicine. New York: McGraw-Hill, 1994; 13:1692– 1698.

* Wobig M, Dickhut A, Maier R et al. Viscosupplementation with hylan G– F 20: A 26– week controlled trial of efficacy and safety in the osteoarthritic knee. Clin Ther 1998; 20:410– 423.

* Creamer P, Sharif M, George E, et al. Intraarticular hyaluronic acid in osteoarthritis of the knee: An investigation into mechanisms of action. Osteoarthritis and Cartilage, 2; 133– 140, 1994.

* Listrat V, Ayral X, Patarnello F et al. evaluation of the potential structure modifying activity of hyaluronan (hyalgan) in osteoarthritis of the knee. Osteoarthritis and Cartilage. 1997; 5:153– 160.

* Felson DT, Zhang Y, Anthony JM, Naimark A, Anderson JJ. Weight loss reduces the risk for symptomatic osteoarthritis in women. The Framingham Study. Ann Intern Med 1992, 116(7):535– 539. 57. Alpiner NM, Oh TN, Brander VA. Rehabilitation in joint and connective tissue diseases. SAE Study Guide 1995, 76(55) 532.

* VanBaar ME, Assendelft WJ, Dekker J et al. Effectiveness of exercise therapy in patients with osteoarthritis of the hip or knee: a systematic review of randomized clinical trials. J Rheumatol 1998; 25(12); 2432– 2439.

* Nordemar R, Ekblom B, Zachrisson L et al. Physical training in rheumatoid arthritis: A controlled long-term study. I. Functional capacity and general attitudes. Scand J Rheum 1981; 10:17– 23.

* Hicks SE. Exercise in patients with inflammatory arthritis and connective tissue disease. Rheum Dis Clinics NA 1990; 16(4):845.

* Clark SR, Burckhardt CS, Bennett RM. Exercise for prevention and treatment of illness. In Exercise for prevention and treatment of illness.

* Basmajian JV and Wolf SL. In: Gerber LH, Hicks JE (eds.), Therapeutic Exercise, 5th edition. Baltimore: Williams and Wilkins, 1990; 340.

* Herbison GJ, Ditunno Jr, Jaweed MM. Muscle atrophy in rheumatoid arthritis. J Rheumatol 1987; S15(14):78– 81.

* Lefebvre JC, KeefeFJ, Affleck G et al. The relationship of arthritis self-efficacy to daily pain, daily mood, and daily pain coping in rheumatoid arthritis patients. Pain 1999; 80:425– 435.

* Parker JC, Smarr KL, Buckelew SP et al. Effects of stress management on clinical outcomes in rheumatoid arthritis. Arthritis Rheum 1995; 38:1807– 1818.

* Williams J, Harvey J, Tannenbaum H. Use of superficial heat versus ice for the rheumatoid arthritic shoulder: A pilot study. Physiotherapy Canada 38:8– 13, 1986.

* Green J, McKenna F, Redfern EJ, Chamberlain MA: Home exercises are as effective as outpatient hydrotherapy for osteoarthritis of the hip. Br J Rheumatol 32:812– 815, 1993.

* Mainardi CL, Walter JM, Spiegel PK, et al. Rheumatoid arthritis: Failure of daily heat therapy to affect its progression. Arch Phys Med Rehabil 1979:60(9); 390– 393.

* Hashish I, Harvey W, Harris M. Antiinflammatory effects of ultrasound therapy: evidence for major placebo effect. Br J Rheumatol 25:77– 81, 1986.

* Oosterveld FGJ, Rasker JJ< Jacobs JWG, Overmars HJA. The effect of local heat and cold therapy on the intraarticular and skin

surface temperature of the knee. Arthritis Rheum 1992; 35:146–151.

* Kumar VN, Redford JB. Transcutaneous nerve stimulation in rheumatoid arthritis. Arch Phys Med Rehabil 63:75– 78, 1987.

* Hayes KW. Physical Modalities. In: Wegener ST, Belza BL, Gall EP (eds.), Clinical Care in the Rheumatic Diseases. Atlanta: American College of Rheumatology, 1996: 79– 82.

* Partridge REH, Duthie JJR. Controlled trial of the effect of complete immobilization of the joints in rheumatoid arthritis. Ann Rheum Dis 22:91– 99, 1963.

* Gault SJ, Spyker JM: Beneficial effects of immobilization of joints in rheumatoid arthritis and related arthritidities: A splint study using sequencial analysis. Arthritis Rheum 12:34– 44, 1969.

* Boden SD. Rheumatoid arthritis of the cervical spine. Surgical decision making based on predictors of paralysis and recovery. Spine 1994; 19(20):2275– 2280.

* Goldberg, VM, Figgie HE, Inglis AE, Figgie MP. Current concepts review: Total elbow arthroplasty. J Bone Joint Surg 1988; 70– A:778– 783. Jolly SL, Ferlic DC, Clayton ML, Dennis DA, Stringer EA. Swanson silicone arthroplasty of wrist in rheumatoid arthritis: A long-term follow-up. J Hand Surg 1992:17:142– 149.

* Monga, Trilok (Editor); Grabois, Martin (Editor). Pain Management in Rehabilitation.

New York, NY, USA: Demos Medical Publishing, 2002. p 232.

http://site.ebrary.com/lib/westthames/Doc?id=10118500&ppg=24

www.ingramcontent.com/pod-product-compliance
Lightning Source LLC
Chambersburg PA
CBHW060620210326
41520CB00010B/1407